Writing for Wellness

A Prescription for Healing

Julie Davey

Idyll Arbor

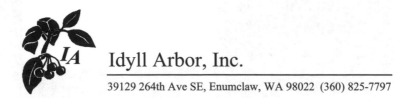

Idyll Arbor, Inc.

39129 264th Ave SE, Enumclaw, WA 98022 (360) 825-7797

ISBN: 9781882883677

Printed in the United States of America

All author's profits from this book will be donated to City of Hope.

Library of Congress Cataloging-in-Publication Data

Davey, Julie.
  Writing for wellness : a prescription for healing / Julie Davey.
      p. cm.
   ISBN-13: 978-1-882883-67-7 (alk. paper)
   1. Graphotherapy. 2. Creative writing--Therapeutic use. 3. Cancer--Patients--Rehabilitation. I. Title.
   RC489.W75D38 2007
   616.89'1--dc22

                                    2007024683

To Bob

my husband, my mentor, my inspiration

Contents

Each chapter contains writing samples, writing lessons and writing prompts to help the reader begin to heal and achieve wellness.

Getting on With Your Life

Compassionate Outcomes

One Family's Cancer Saga

Foreword

While we all recognize that words can readily help or harm, this volume is testimony to the healing and restorative capacity of language. There are so many elements of a person's life beyond his or her control, or even influence, that it is refreshing and liberating to realize that written self-expression can be a powerful reservoir of comfort.

Everyone associated with the seriously ill patient or someone who has suffered great loss or tragedy — health-care providers, friends, and family — instinctively understands the need for comfort and, within the limits of our collective capacity, we try to provide it. However, inevitably, even the most caring of us can become spiritually exhausted and depleted of compassion. Consequently, each person in contact with the patient has need of healing and restoration.

There are a great many sources of renewal — religion, literature, music, and companionship, to name a few. This volume vividly demonstrates that a potent source of restoration of hope, compassion, and care comes through the act of writing. The simple, profound act of written self-expression is, in itself, a remarkable miracle.

As a medical oncologist for more than 35 years, I have cared for thousands of patients. I have seen the toll exacted by cancer on patients, families, friends, and caregivers. I have also been impressed by how effective this writing program has been and can be. I recommend it to you, the reader, as one worthwhile outlet for the universal condition of caring intensely about our fellow man.

Michael A. Friedman, M.D.
President and CEO
City of Hope National Medical Center

vii

◀ ◀ ◆ ▶ ▶

As a child, I enjoyed reading the dictionary. I delighted in words and their derivation.

As a physician, I learned long ago in medical school the power of words, as descriptors (Where exactly is the lesion?), and as diagnoses, without which there is no appropriate therapy.

As a mother of toddlers, I learned the importance for a child of being able to articulate feelings ("Matthew, don't cry. Tell me what's wrong. Use words; words are your friends.")

Now, as I have followed Professor Davey's writing classes, I have seen the healing power of words, used as precise tools, even as weapons by patients in their battle against cancer.

Professor Davey has taught her students to think and to articulate. For them writing has been more than an intellectual exercise.

By giving of herself and sharing her own integrity and loving kindness, she has inspired her students to reach deep down inside themselves, to feel, and to heal.

I am proud to have had a part of this experience that has helped so many.

Lucille A. Leong, M.D.
Associate Director of Clinical Affairs
Division of Medical Oncology
City of Hope National Medical Center

Acknowledgements

First and foremost, there would be no book at all without my husband Bob's editing of the manuscript. Every contributor and reader owes him a debt of gratitude, as do I.

Thank you to Dr. Michael Friedman, President and CEO of City of Hope National Medical Center, for continuing to support Writing for Wellness classes on the campus and for endorsing them as an effective form of therapy.

Writing this book has been an honor. I have had the privilege of meeting hundreds of inspirational students who initially attended my classes to learn writing techniques to help them heal, but who instead taught me innumerable life lessons. As we continue to interact, I witness your courage, your determination, your tenacity, and your direct role in battling disease. You are my heroes.

Without City of Hope staff members Linda Baginski and Jeanne Lawrence there would have been no Writing for Wellness class. Shirley Otis-Green and Lynn Palmer have also paved the way, ensuring success. All have attended the classes and have their inspirational writing included in this book, along with those of Marilyn Rhodes, RN, who has also counseled many of my own friends and relatives. The stirring writings of City of Hope's Annie Watson also appear in the book and reflect how she encourages, calms, inspires, and soothes patients who arrive for treatments each day. Thanks to Anna Escobosa, a colon-cancer survivor, who called CBS News and convinced them to do a story about our class. We were on the evening news and I was named Woman of the Week in Los Angeles.

Thank you, Dr. Lucille Leong, my oncologist, for your holistic view of medicine that includes both healing me and also sending other patients of yours to be helped by the Writing for Wellness class experience. Thank you, Dr. James Andersen, my surgeon, for giving me my life back after you expertly performed the 12-hour bilateral tram-flap procedure that restored me physically and psychologically. Thank you, Dr. Janice DaVolio, my dermatologist, for your talent and dedication in keeping my raging psoriasis from taking over my life. All three of these very special physicians have dedicated their lives to making dramatic and positive differences in the quality of life of their patients.

Thank you, Mary Ellen Lepionka, for encouraging me to continue the quest for publication. Thanks to Bill Durkee, Bill Matteson, and Joan Smith for reading various drafts of the manuscript and for believing in the value of this book. Elizabeth Terry, Rick Myers, Chakib Sambar, and Dr. Lois Neil also deserve thanks for serving as substitute teachers over the years and inspiring the Writing for Wellness students.

Thank you to all the contributors, those who took a chance to write from their hearts about what they were experiencing as a result of cancer or other tragedies in their lives. You did not have to share your stories but chose to do so to help others feel less isolated as they, too, try to heal.

For his belief in the book, his professional editing, and creative formatting, as well as his dedication to the project, I thank Tom Blaschko, president of Idyll Arbor

Heartfelt thanks to my former Fullerton College student, graphic artist Vince Williams, who designed the cover. Special thanks to photographer Markie Ramirez who captured the spirit of the class she also attends.

Special thanks and admiration go to Christine Pechera, Elizabeth Terry, Steve Rom, Jerome Williams, and Charles Fell whose tenacity and faith continue to transform the gossamer thread between life and death into a steel rod to lift themselves and others into the light.

Introduction

Cancer and other life-threatening illnesses and tragedies affect us all, no matter our age, our position in life, or our education. We all know someone in our family or among our friends and co-workers who has suffered. And sometimes, for millions of us, we have been touched very personally. According to statistics, one out of three people will be diagnosed with some form of cancer during their lifetime. For those who have not experienced it directly, there is the unspoken but nagging concern that cancer might pay an unexpected visit one day. This is an unwelcome, but common, bond we share.

Even if you don't have personal experience with cancer, you may have suffered a tragedy or loss in your life — as a victim of child abuse, crime, abandonment, or neglect, or perhaps by losing someone close to you through illness or accident.

In more than five years of teaching expressive writing techniques to cancer patients and those who have experienced a vast array of tragedies, what I have learned is simple: words can help you heal. A doctor can help heal your body, and a psychiatrist or a good friend with a soft shoulder can help heal your spirit. But, focused and directed writing about what you are going through in the depths of your soul provides a unique and sometimes immediate sense of relief. That experience can also be the beginning of a special kind of healing.

I have written this book for many reasons, first to chronicle a unique and continuing class called Writing for Wellness, and next to provide guidelines for you, the reader, to experience the healing process yourself. I also hope to inspire others to start Writing for Wellness classes in small towns and large cities everywhere.

My personal journey with cancer connects me with those of you who are going through diagnosis or treatment now as well as those who have survived both. Since my parents both died from the disease and many of my friends and family members have as well, I can also identify with the caregivers, children, and friends of the patients.

Each chapter in the book begins with some of my personal experiences. Under *Healing Words* my students' writings appear in each chapter, and almost all of the epigraphs (quotations that begin each chapter) are also student-written. *It's Your Turn* ends each chapter and contains ideas and suggestions, a prescription, if you will, for you to use to begin writing your own story. There is also a *Jump Start* section with a sentence or two to help you begin to write.

Throughout the book, I use what we in the teaching profession call the "tell-one, show-one, do-one" method of writing instruction. First, I tell you my experiences through my own writings, next I show you written examples of how others (my students) have expressed themselves on the same topic, and, finally, I ask you to do your own writing on that subject. I find the method to be easy for writers as well as so-called non-writers to follow. Students in my classes who say they used to have trouble getting started discover they can begin writing almost immediately and are eager for the next lesson.

As you go through the writing exercises, listen to your own feelings and guard them. Once you have completed a lesson, there is no need to rush to share a piece of your writing. You may want to wait until you feel very secure with another person. Or you may choose never to share some of the things you write.

Every story starts with the first word.

Enjoy the process.

Part I

Getting Started

Chapter 1

Class Is in Session

You are not your disease.
Cancer does not define you; you define you. It
can never steal your identity or essence. You are
not cancer and cancer is not you.

— Edna Teller

Since 2001, I have been teaching writing to cancer patients, their family members, doctors, nurses, caregivers, and others who may have suffered tragic events in their lives.

Writing for Wellness classes are held at the City of Hope National Cancer Center in Duarte, California, the site Lance Armstrong, one of the world's most famous cancer survivors, chose to start his 2004 cross-country bicycle tour for cancer awareness.

My experience began a few days following 9/11 when I was walking on the City of Hope grounds to an appointment at my oncologist's office. I witnessed a group of very young children, some only five or six years old, dressed in their slippers and pajamas. On that clear, warm fall day

5

they were in a single line following a young man in his 20s, who wore a volunteer's identification badge.

As they walked around the medical center's grounds outside its pediatric oncology building, they skipped, clapped their hands, and waved their arms. Each tiny child had a bald head from chemotherapy and wore a surgical mask for protection against germs, obviously young leukemia patients on an exercise field trip from their hospital beds. While their leader counted out, "One! Two!" the children kept time. Some marched in military style; others bobbed their heads to imaginary music. All of them seemed to be enjoying their outing.

As the children passed by, I felt a tug at my heartstrings. They were so young to have a major disease, yet they seemed to be coping with what life had dealt them. As I watched, I also realized that the volunteer was doing something significant, selfless.

At that defining moment, I vowed to do something myself to help other people. I had never consistently volunteered anywhere before. Over the years, I had occasionally taught Sunday school, tutored underprivileged teens prior to their SAT tests, and helped with various civic projects when my husband was mayor of our small town.

But this was different. This time I knew I wanted to try to make a continuing and significant difference in people's lives. Following that young volunteer's example, I was determined to give something back.

Less than a week earlier, two hours after the World Trade Center Towers collapsed, I was in my classroom facing 30 journalism students at Fullerton College as we all tried to make sense of what had just happened. I told them that we should promise to devote ourselves, in any way we could, to ridding the world of evil.

With tears in my own eyes, I stared at their tear-stained faces. I was barely able to speak.

"We all have skills," I told them, my voice cracking. "Use yours; help somebody. Make a difference."

My students, ranging from 18 to more than 60 years old, nodded in agreement. I told them I was convinced that volunteering could help us begin to heal from the tragedy.

Over the years my parents, who were both very generous with their time and money, told me that when bad things happened not to feel sorry for myself but to take action because, "There's always someone worse off than you."

Recalling their words, I asked myself what I could do immediately.

That day during my appointment, I revealed to Dr. Lucille Leong my deep desire to volunteer. She encouraged me and gave me some names and numbers for contacts at City of Hope.

I had seen volunteers driving cancer patients around in golf carts from building to building on the 112-acre campus to assist those who had trouble walking to their doctors' appointments. I could do that.

Or, perhaps I should offer my assistance in the public relations office since I knew how to write news releases. Maybe I could publicize new cancer treatments to get the word out to those who needed help. My mind was searching to find a place for me.

Driving home I continued to think about what I had to offer. Then suddenly, it came to me. I realized I could teach writing to my fellow cancer patients/survivors and their caregivers to help them express what they were going through.

That afternoon I called the Patient and Family Resource Desk and outlined my plan. I explained I was a two-time survivor, having had breast cancer in 1984 and again in 1996, telling them I was also a full-time college writing professor. I added what I had discovered firsthand, that when people write about tragedies in their lives, they feel better.

Then, with the assistance of Linda Baginski, herself a breast cancer survivor, and another cancer survivor, Jeanne Lawrence, and Shirley Otis-Green, all part of the Patient Services team, we named the class "Writing for Wellness" and sessions were scheduled almost immediately.

If there was any red tape, they had sliced right through it.

The time and place were set and flyers were posted. As we had outlined, the class would be open to cancer patients, their family members and caregivers, and all staff members at City of Hope. The flyer also said the class would be open to anyone who had experienced a major illness or tragedy. We stressed that no previous writing experience was necessary.

I became excited about the prospect of the class, but I wasn't sure if anyone would actually show up.

The room I was assigned for the class (shown on the back cover) instantly created a positive atmosphere. Named the "Hope Village Comedy Theatre," it is a small room with all its walls colorfully painted with almost life-sized caricatures of comedians, actors, and cartoon characters. Lucy and Desi, Laurel and Hardy, Bart Simpson, Garfield, and many others smile at all who enter. I could not help smiling back.

The room had two pianos, a small stage, and lots of comfortable chairs.

Strongly believing in the power of effective group dynamics, I immediately moved some tables and chairs into a horseshoe shape with the opening facing my chair. That way, everyone would be able to write and to see everyone else. I did not want to lecture or stand at a podium. I wanted no barriers between my "students" and me. I wanted to be on the same level as them. After all, we were all in this cancer thing together.

I later learned that there were weekly Bingo games held there for the pediatric patients and their family members, and it was also the site of many adult support-group meetings. The room exuded positive energy.

My first class was in the evening. I set the time from 6:30 to 8:00, realizing that many cancer patients still had jobs as did their family members and caregivers. I also wanted people from the general public to be able to attend after work. I brought coffee, soft drinks, and desserts.

As I left my house with the food, plus a coffee maker, cups, plates, plastic utensils, and a tablecloth, my husband, Bob, teased, "What are you teaching anyway, cooking?"

Throughout my years of teaching high school and college, I have been known as a "feeder," bringing snacks to most of my classes, especially when overseeing the late-night production of campus newspapers. Bob had seen this all before.

My journalism students, notoriously hungry and frequently broke, always ran to help me as I negotiated my way to class with shopping bags stuffed with food they would soon be devouring. But that night at City of Hope as I unloaded my car, I felt odd, unsure of myself.

Over the years, I had taught thousands of students ranging from high school sophomores to senior citizens taking college courses, but I felt this class would be like none other.

Then, suddenly, as I was setting up the room and refreshments, I became very nervous. My palms started to sweat; a sense of dread swept over me.

What had I gotten myself into? What if the cancer patients or their family members broke into tears and sobbed? What if someone who had suffered a great tragedy felt worse after coming to my class? I wasn't a trained psychologist. How arrogant of me to think I could actually help someone in such a simple manner, "Writing for Wellness" indeed.

I stared at the clock. It was 6:25. Five minutes to go. I wanted to run out of the door. Then a short Hispanic man in his late 60s who spoke with a slight accent walked in. He was smiling and shook hands enthusiastically. He picked up some refreshments, sat down, and opened a notebook. He had his pen ready. He talked very rapidly.

"I'm Bob. I had pancreatic cancer. I should be dead, but I beat it! Plus, I'm a diabetic, too!" he told me proudly. "Now, I want to write poetry."

I sighed and immediately felt at ease. Then, as eight more people showed up, carried desserts and drinks to the tables, and sat down facing me, I realized I might be able to handle it after all. They all looked eager and friendly.

As soon as everyone was seated, I asked the participants to introduce themselves and tell about their experiences with cancer or other diseases or tragedies. I wondered if people would be hesitant to share that information with total strangers. They were not. I had to choose from among several raised hands as we started to meet one another.

Joan, 60s, who had almost no hair, talked about battling breast cancer. Marilyn, 50s, a registered nurse with daily and often stressful interactions with cancer patients, revealed how her job affected her. Milynne, 30s, with a slight jaundiced look and very little energy despite the sweet smile on her face, told us she had liver cancer, but she was determined to write about what she was going through. Ramona, 60s, fighting cancer for 12 years said she wanted to thank her daughter for helping her. Tony, late 40s, was not a cancer patient. He had come to the class because he had lost his only child, a 27-year-old son in an accident. Tony said he wanted to see if writing about the tragedy would help him find some peace.

On it went. Some were patients, some were family members, and some were health-care professionals. Others had seen the flyer and thought the class might help them deal with some catastrophe in their lives.

One thread tied us all together — the desire to write about our experiences.

As each person spoke, I began to see what a great need there was for such a class, an outlet for those holding in the stress that dealing with cancer or any other serious medical situation or tragedy can create. These people needed to talk, to write, and to interact with others who were going through similar experiences. I became aware of how intently the students were listening to one another's stories and I completely forgot about my nervousness.

Following their introductions, I gave mine. I told them I had been a college writing professor for more than 15 years and had written many newspaper and magazine articles, one published novel, and, like everyone else who lived near Hollywood, a couple of unsold screenplays. But, when I said I was also a two-time breast cancer survivor, I could see visible changes in their faces. They knew we had a lot in common.

I wasn't just another teacher.

And from my experiences in that room, I continue to realize that it isn't just another class.

Healing Words

Participants in the class share their writings, their fears, and their dreams. In this section throughout the book, you will share those with them. As you read what other cancer patients and people who have gone through tragedies have written, you may also find ideas and ways to express what you have experienced.

Donna Logan, 36, an elementary school teacher, was diagnosed twice with an aggressive form of breast cancer. She had two mastectomies and was healing when the cancer returned. In a desperate attempt to save her life, she left for North Carolina for clinical-trial treatments at Duke University Medical Center. Family members pitched in to care for her three small daughters left behind. Donna's husband, Matt, a local high school football coach, traveled between the two states, dividing his time as best he could. Prior to leaving for her treatment, Donna and her mother, Theda Clark, attended Writing for Wellness class.

Everyone in her family was affected by Donna's cancer, including her 10-year-old daughter Lindsey who wrote the following:

As Brave As a Lion

As brave as a lion, as tough as a bear,
She fights even when she loses her hair.
That chemo just won't go away,
But she still fights it every day.
She's had cancer three times now,
And it has everyone wondering how,
Through all of this, she remains calm.
I'm proud to say that she's my Mom.

— Lindsey Logan

Charles Fell, 60s, a deputy State Attorney General in Hawaii, was unable to move. He lay completely still in his sterile hospital room, his wife, Elena, in gown, gloves, and mask beside him. She had heard about Writing for Wellness class and had come to the Hope Village kitchen one morning before my class to ask me if I ever made "house calls." Her eyes were pleading and I had no idea what lay ahead.

I immediately agreed to meet her in Charles' room inside the six-story hospital. When I arrived, nurses told me to wash my hands, put on a hospital gown, gloves, and a mask for the visit. Immediately upon entering his room, I could see that it was only Charles' body that was immobilized. His spirit and mind were very much intact. He greeted me, thanked me for coming, and asked if he could recite a poem for me. For several minutes, lying motionless, he recited a wonderful poem he had composed that, when printed out, would have been more than a page of writing. I got tears in my eyes as I saw him, only able to move his mouth, yet he was eloquent, clearly in love with language. And, as he recited his descriptive and lyrical poem, writing was also obviously helping him cope.

He was, I learned later, at the lowest physical point possible before a transplant can take place, probably as close to death as he had ever been. He would begin the transplant in a matter of hours. If it worked, he would live. If it did not, he would die. Period. After his bone marrow transplant, Charles, still wearing a surgical mask, sat in the classroom area I reserve for "masked bandits," apart from the other patients who may have germs or bacteria. Even months after transplant, patients still have to be careful.

A few weeks later, Charles wheeled in again, this time under his own power. When I last saw him in person, he was ready to go back to Hawaii and he was walking and waving his arms in delight. The transplant had taken. Charles had made it. In the following poem, which Charles composed at night and dictated to Elena the following morning, he describes how he and Elena dealt with his cancer diagnosis.

Cancer's Montage

A tear on the plate,
And I'm up and out; I'm late.
A tear on a plate,
And my wife ponders my fate.

A tear in a cup,
And we ask ourselves how much?
A tear in a cup,
And our fingertips touch.

A pull on a sleeve,
And a phone call comes.
A pull on a sleeve,
And she whispers she loves me.

A gaze at the night sky,
And the stars are still there.
A gaze at the night sky,
And we ask ourselves why?

A tear on the bed,
When the Bible is read.
A tear on the bed,
But nothing much ever said.

— Charles F. Fell

Robert Prado, 68, the father of seven children, had finally worked enough years to earn his retirement from a major glass company. He thought life would be sweet from then on, no schedules or pressures, just enjoyment. Then things changed. Robert writes about how a simple request from a grandchild helped give him strength to fight and ultimately beat the almost always deadly pancreatic cancer that had nearly consumed him.

A Thousand Times Yes

Retirement at last!
Now I can enjoy life more.
Then the doctor says, "Cancer!"
After surgery, radiation, chemotherapy,

And pills, pills, and more pills,
All this is making me more ill,
More ill than the cancer.
A lot of bad days and a few better days.
On the bad days I feel like giving up.
Then a good day comes along and I feel better.
On one bad day when I felt like giving up,
A small voice said, "Grandpa, could you tie my shoes?"
And I said, "Why yes, precious, a hundred times yes.
In fact a thousand times yes!"

— **Robert Prado**

It's Your Turn

On a piece of paper or at your computer begin to describe your experience with a life-threatening disease, a major loss, or a tragedy. You may be or have been a patient, a spouse, a friend, a family member, or a caregiver. Write about how you feel now or have felt during the crisis. Include as many details as you can. Journalists use the word "when" if they have trouble getting a story started. The three dots indicate places for your words.

Jump Start

When I first was told ... had ... I felt ... After a while, I felt ... and as time progressed, my emotions changed to ...

Continue to write and include answers to these questions:

Is your condition/situation a continuing one?

How does/did the experience affect you emotionally?

How do you feel now? Give details.

Did anything positive come from the experience? Explain.

Remember, you have an interesting story to tell. Don't leave out important details. You'll get the idea. After you describe the events, stop to see how you feel. Did writing help you? Explain how. Sometimes people experience a physical sense of relief; others say it is simply mental peace of mind. Telling your story may release your stress or simply allow you to put the events into perspective. When you are through, place your writing into a personal notebook or computer folder.

Save your writing. It tells the story of what you are going through or what you have already experienced. As you read this book, you will be guided through specific steps in *It's Your Turn* to help you heal by writing.

Chapter 2

Personal Experience

*Fear of an early death is not fear of death itself.
It is fear of being forgotten, of disappearing into that
blackness of forever*

— Christine Pechera

That first night of class, I told my students about my own experience with writing for wellness.

My father, a retired florist in his 60s, had contracted aplastic anemia. It was determined that he had been exposed to DDT over many years when he was manager of a large wholesale floral company. The doctors told him DDT exposure had been identified as a major cause of his condition and that he needed an immediate bone marrow transplant. That was impossible because, at that time, only siblings could donate the marrow and his older sister was too ill to serve as his donor.

At the time of my father's exposure, the late 1940s and into the 1950s, apparently no one realized that if DDT killed bugs, it might also kill people. Later, Rachel Carson wrote about its deadly effects in her book *Silent Spring*. Today, the substance is banned in the U.S. and most other countries.

Immediately after he was diagnosed and my mother (Mozelle), my brother (Lynn), and I were told that his condition was terminal, I found myself desperate to say many things to him. I tried to talk to him in person but it didn't work. Words caught in my throat and I ended up crying and, I'm sure, making him feel very sad in the process. We Americans, as a culture, sometimes have a hard time putting our emotions into words when we are face to face. It can seem strained and awkward for everyone concerned.

My parents were not ones who often said, "I love you!" to each other or to my brother or me. People today, at least in California, now say that routinely, sometimes to near strangers. Times were a bit more formal in the 1950s when I was growing up. The love era of the sixties allowed many to express more freely those once-private emotions.

My parents' actions always showed their love; my brother and I knew how they felt. I assumed my father probably knew how I felt, too. But somehow when a person is terminally ill, all of those emotions rise to the surface. If the opportunity to speak or to write is not taken, then it is truly lost forever.

I needed to write him a letter.

With pen and paper I told him how much he meant to me, how much I loved him, and how grateful I was to have had him for my father. I sobbed as I composed the letter and had to recopy it because of my tear stains. It was my first experience with the healing power of writing.

I felt greatly relieved after I finished the letter. I wrote things I had wanted to tell him for years and never did. I took some time to go back and revise the letter until I felt it was ready to send.

Here is part of my letter:

Dear Daddy,

... other memories are of taking bouquets of flowers you gave me to Mrs. Briscoe, my third-grade teacher at Steele School. I realize now that, by giving those special gifts to her, you were showing me that teachers were special people — people you held in high esteem. I know that had a big influence on my choice of careers. No other kid in my class ever brought such large or expensive bouquets to her. Others might bring a rose or a bunch of sweet peas from their gardens, but not a real bouquet wrapped in green florist's paper with a package of Flora-life inside. This made me special to my teacher and she'd often say, "You're so lucky to have such a nice father!" I knew that.

The last memory and probably the most important one was how you treated Mom all those years. We could always tell you loved her, and continue to. You don't always remember Valentine's Day or even her birthday without some coaching, but you show your love every day. You do it by being there for her, enjoying being together, and helping in so many small ways to give her a good life. That kindness does not go unnoticed by her or us. Lynn and I could always tell you loved each other and still do. It was nice to come from that kind of home. So many people never see or experience true love in their lifetimes.

Thank you for loving me. I love you, too. Julie

I mailed the letter to Colorado Springs. My mother telephoned to tell me how much he cherished it, rereading it numerous times. And later, from his hospital bed where he spent his last days, he choked back tears to thank me personally for writing it.

After he died, as I left the hospital, I noticed the structure itself stood as an ominous symbol. I had a hard time even looking at the building without feeling deep sadness. Again I wrote, that time to myself, my words reflecting a bitterness at losing my dear father and leaving him there inside.

Memorial Hospital

The town's largest building is a massive concrete structure,
Towering over small bungalows of wood and plaster.
Inside, antiseptic people scurry with special instructions,
Individualized diets and powerful potions to save, nay prolong,
The lives of those confined, those labeled, "The Terminals,"
Who are talked to in unnatural, too-soothing tones about
Tomorrow and Future when those locked in their beds by weakness
Know that Today is all there is.
Relatives with eyes sore from tears held in,
Sit all night, counting breaths; others go home but do not sleep.
Telephone calls break the night's silence, making knees weak
And stomachs churn, although "expected."
Still, in morning's light, coldly and monolithic
The large structure remains,
The only tombstone not in the cemetery.

— **Julie Bolger Davey**

(Edward Lynn Bolger died at age 67.)

Healing Words

Allison Anderson was 22 when her father was diagnosed with cancer. When I first met Allison, I had no idea what emotions she was holding inside. She looked and acted much like other young students of mine at the local community college. She was taking Journalism 101 along with about 25 others who came directly from work for the weekly three-hour class. They came in carrying large drink cups and sandwiches for the 6:00 to 9:00 p.m. seminar, all trying to get a degree while working full time. I never minded them eating. None of them talked much for the first half hour or so, winding down from their jobs and the stress of freeway traffic. But, Allison, more quiet than most, was never one to wave her hand to be called on or to call attention to herself. She seemed distracted, in another world. One evening, I gave an assignment to the group to write a "nostalgia" article in which they were to recall a special moment from their childhood. When I read Allison's words, I realized why she had been so quiet.

Many and Many a Year Ago...

As a little girl, my favorite thing to do was to read poetry with my father. Before I could even spell my own name, Dad would read me poems about war, loyalty, friendship, and love. He would call to me, "Ali, do you want to bring me my books?"

Beaming, I would run to his bookshelf and grab the worn-out books and carefully bring them to him. I would curl up beside him and pretend I could follow along on the page as he read aloud.

"Daddy, now read Annabel Lee, okay?" I would plead.

And he would begin.

"It was many and many a year ago, in a kingdom by the sea..."

I would sit up with him until I fell asleep and like magic, I would wake up the next morning in my own bed.

When I was able to read myself, we would take turns. He would choose a poem and then I would. If I would mispronounce a word, he would gently correct me and we would discuss its meaning at great length.

Like all little girls feel about their fathers, I thought my Dad was the smartest man alive. But, my teenage years saw a waning of our recitals. I would much rather hang out with my friends than hang out with Dad and read. He never mentioned the change. It would be years before we read together again.

Two years ago, my father was diagnosed with cancer. It was growing from his jaw. A couple of months after his diagnosis, we were told that there was nothing more that could be done. His doctors told him to go home and enjoy the rest of the few weeks he had left. It would be a strange reversal for me to go from the one who was always cared for, to becoming the caregiver.

Thankfully, my mother forced him to get a second opinion. City of Hope would perform the surgery that would extend his life — the removal of his jaw.

The whole family was on pins and needles during his 18-hour surgery. It was successful. Afterwards, only my mother, sister, and I were allowed to see him. I sat down on his bed in the Intensive Care Unit and opened a book.

"It was many and many a year ago, in a kingdom by the sea..."

— Allison Anderson

(A year after Allison wrote this in my class, her father died.)

It's Your Turn

Words are sometimes all we have. Speaking them in person is often too painful. We choke up; we don't seem to get them to come out in the way we intended. Writing them down may make us shed tears in the process, but afterwards we feel comforted knowing that we have said what we wanted to say to the person we loved.

Jump Start

Dear   ...
As I look back over my life to this point, I remember a time when ...

I feel fortunate because without you ...

Don't worry about spelling or grammar. Realize that you can go back later and fix those things or add additional facts, feelings, and details. Get started now. Think of this as a work in progress. Take time to write today and tomorrow and the next day. Then, as appropriate, send or deliver the letter. If the person has already passed away, you may want to read it aloud as if you are addressing them. Or, read it to a living relative of theirs. Then, put it safely away in a special place and read it from time to time when you think of that special person in your life. Your words will keep the person alive through your memories.

Chapter 3

Violet's Story

We never really die, do we?
We live on in the hearts and spirits
of those we touch.
My grandmother lives on through her writing.
— Vivianne Wightman

It was an older and wiser person who taught me the most valuable lessons I have ever learned about how writing can provide comfort after tragedy and illness and even create peace of mind when the end of life is near. Violet was the model student for Writing for Wellness. Here is her story:

Sitting on a Cloud

When 91-year-old Violet Wightman walked into my writing class at Fullerton College and proceeded to introduce herself as a friend of both Sergei Rachmaninoff and Amelia Earhart, I was dumbfounded.

First, I didn't actually believe her, and second, I could think of no response but a rather unenthusiastic, "That's nice."

I immediately pointed to the student next to her to continue with the first-day introductions.

Violet instantly recognized my skepticism and at the next class brought a yellowed newspaper clipping and photo showing her with the famous aviatrix. I didn't dare ask about Rachmaninoff.

So, when she announced that he personally wrote a polka for her when she was a world-famous concert pianist, I never doubted it for a second.

She had come to my class as a frail, hard-of-hearing woman who had many health problems, but she didn't want to discuss them publicly. She wanted to write.

Over the next several years, Violet came to my classes. She became a fixture. She was talented, humorous, and energetic. She was always immaculately dressed, sitting among students in their torn blue jeans and sweatshirts. She still holds the record at Fullerton College, an institution with 22,000 students, as the oldest ever enrolled. She also remains my all-time favorite student.

She was quick-witted and sarcastic, a combination that sometimes took the other students by surprise.

"I don't have to do what you say!" she loudly announced in class one day when I was assigning what she thought was unnecessary homework. "Remember, I'm older than you!" Then, she winked.

Her tanned, pierced, and tattooed 19-year-old California classmates howled with delight.

She would often refer to me as a "slave driver" after I assigned what she felt were overly difficult writing projects. But, at each class session Violet would smile gratefully at me from her seat in the front row. We understood one another without words.

She was, indeed, a model student, bringing in parts of her

sometimes racy in-progress novels, stories of her childhood in the Arizona Territory before its statehood, as well as some of her unforgettable and lyrical poetry.

Other students had taken my freelance writing class to learn to sell short articles to magazines and newspapers, hoping for some needed cash to help with the rent on their apartment. But Violet had her own immediate dream, a dream to see her words in print before she died.

Then, when she was 96, she developed breast cancer and she saw her dream to be published as urgent. After she told the class about her diagnosis and her surgery, I revealed that I, too, was a breast cancer survivor. Violet and I became even closer.

"We really are like sisters, you know," she said, smiling. "But, just remember I'm the older one!"

Many times in class I felt that she was actually my teacher and I was her student. As she talked about growing up in the horse-and-buggy days in Globe, Arizona, and then traveling around the world as a concert pianist, I knew she had far more life experiences than I would ever have. She had also lost her husband in a car accident in Europe and had raised four children as a single mother.

Her life had not been easy.

"I want my poems published," she announced to me one day after class. "I want to leave them to my family. I'll need your help." I learned later that she had also written musical backgrounds for her poems and had often sung them to her grandchildren.

As her health continued to deteriorate, one of Violet's classmates, Ellen Mortensen, a registered nurse, volunteered to type Violet's poems onto a floppy disk so they could be more easily accessed by a publisher or printer.

I knew that a professional publisher was out of the question for Violet's poems. She simply didn't have the months it might take to try to find an agent or to query a mainstream publisher. In fact, it seemed she had so little time left that I wondered if her dream would ever be realized. Cancer was consuming her before our eyes.

One day Violet asked to address my entire class. She stood and faced the students, holding onto my desk to steady herself. She was always stylishly dressed and her hair was nicely done. From her days as a globetrotting performer, she also knew how to command an audience's attention. She paused to be sure everyone was listening.

"You know that even though the doctors tell me I'm going to die, I am not going to!" she said with determination, her voice strong with resolve.

We were immobilized by her announcement. We knew she was getting weaker every day, yet she insisted on attending each class session even though she often seemed to be in great pain. To ensure her safety as she walked on the campus, her family hired a nurse to accompany her. Violet seemed to resent the lack of independence, but she also seemed to know she needed the assistance.

Although she often surprised us, none of us was prepared for her words that day.

"No, I tell you, I'm not going to die!" she said. "I'm just going to sit up in the sky on a cloud and watch you all. Think of me up there whenever you see one of those big white fluffy ones. That'll be me."

Violet's clear blue eyes stared at each of us as we wiped away tears. As she started to slowly walk back to her seat a few feet away, she turned and gently patted my hand. I could barely speak when I tried to start the day's lesson.

After class that day Ellen and I took the diskette with Violet's poems on it to the college print shop and asked the instructors for help.

"We need these poems printed as a book and we need it done immediately; she doesn't have long."

The printing instructors and their students began working feverishly to get the book of poems ready for print. Within a few days we got an urgent call. They needed our immediate input.

"We're almost ready to print, but we don't have a title and we don't know what color the cover should be!"

Without hesitation, I answered, "Make the cover violet, and call the book *Sitting on a Cloud.*"

A few weeks later when Violet saw her book, she was delighted. Then, as she did with many things, she decided it could have been better. She liked to control things and we had made some important decisions without her input.

"That's Julie's idea for a title, not mine!" she grumbled to the class. "And, I've always hated violet — both the color and my name."

Then she smiled. "I love my book, though," she said with pride as she gave each of us an autographed copy with personal notes thanking each student and me for our support.

After Violet's book of poems came out, I called the *Los Angeles Times* to ask for a reporter to be sent to class. He came and he wrote an in-depth article about her, especially about her past as a well-known pianist who was indeed friends with both Rachmaninoff and Earhart. The piece ran with a color photo of Violet with her classmates.

Many Los Angeles area friends of Violet's with whom she had lost contact over the years, read the article and telephoned her, asking for copies of her book.

Her family was overwhelmed. Violet's dream had been realized. Her words had helped her, and she had left her family a priceless gift. She seemed at peace.

She began cloud-sitting less than a month later.

Healing Words

Here is one of Violet's poems.

Dancing Water

Oh, to be merry dancing water
In a fountain
Sparkling in the sunlight
Tossing diamonds at the moon.
To know the joy of saucy robins
Bathing in my bosom,
Splashing veils of mist to thirsty flowers,
Liquid song notes to the breeze.
And lest cold winter snows
Should hold me fast,
I would trickle to a brook,
From the brook to a river,
And from the river to the sea.
But, if perchance you were a yellow butterfly
Passing by the fountain,
I would climb upon the first white cloud
That sailed blue skies for home,
And slide down a rainbow through the sky,
And descend upon your outspread wings,
With tender springtime kisses in the rain.
If you were a yellow butterfly.
Oh to be merry dancing water
In a fountain.

— Violet Wightman

Bernice "Bebe" Goetz has been a friend of the Wightman family for more than 40 years and has also consistently attended Writing for Wellness classes. She relates a story repeatedly told to her by Violet in

her advanced years. Violet had been a concert pianist and her husband had been "the dentist to the Hollywood stars," causing them to interact with some of the movie and entertainment industry's wealthiest people, fellow residents of Beverly Hills. On a family trip to France, Violet's husband was killed in an auto accident and she, her son, and one daughter were badly injured. Her world was shattered. Once back home in California, she found herself in need of a steady income to support her and her four children. Buying, repairing, and then selling small rentals seemed to be her answer.

Violet's tiny hands for which Rachmaninoff wrote a special polka were now cleaning, painting, and repairing rental properties to make ends meet. It was a family business and her children were always working, too.

Bebe presents the story in Violet's own words.

Shocking the "Ladies Who Lunch"

My friends in Beverly Hills are so boring. All they do is go to lunch every Thursday, play cards, and gossip. Even after I moved to Fullerton, they kept after me to come up for their Thursday lunches.

I never had time for that.

But one Thursday, I agreed to meet them at a very expensive and exclusive restaurant. All of the ladies were chattering about going shopping, lunches, and cards. I was so bored. Finally, they got around to asking me what I had been doing.

I opened my purse, pulled out a screwdriver, and laid it on the fine linen tablecloth.

They were horrified! (At this point Violet smiled her relishing-the-moment smile as she continued to tell Bebe the story.) Then I pulled out a pair of pliers and laid it down.

One especially shocked lady exclaimed, "Violet, you can't do that in here!"

I proceeded to pull a hammer out of my purse and laid it down, too.

My lady friends were appalled and embarrassed at my crass display of poor etiquette and breeding and continued with their disparaging remarks, gasping in dismay.

I finally said, looking at each of them, "You're still leading a boring life! Well, I'm not and never will!"

It was the last of my Thursday luncheons in Beverly Hills.

— Bernice "Bebe" Goetz

Violet's son, Don, her daughter-in-law, Janine, and her granddaughter, Vivianne, attended Writing for Wellness class to help them heal from Violet's passing. Her granddaughter, who now teaches journalism at Fullerton College, wrote the following:

She Lives On

Writing is one way to celebrate life and its blessings, and to work through its pitfalls and hardships.

I know from my grandmother, Violet. Her stories were an affront to all the hardships and negativity life had dealt her — the early death of her husband and a daughter, being a single mother, and picking up trash and cleaning laundry rooms to make ends meet when her heart and soul are aching to be playing piano and traveling from one grand performance to the next.

In her writings, my grandmother lives on — and so do her precious memories of those she loved.

Violet is always with me, Julie, as she is with you. We never really die, do we? We just live on and on in the hearts and spirits of those we touch.

I am a firm believer that this life is not the end, but that doesn't mean we shouldn't embrace living with every last ounce of fight and passion we can muster. The blessings of life come in sharing our love, our passions, and our hearts with others.

— Vivianne Wightman

It's Your Turn

Violet left her family the gift of words. Write about words you may have received from someone. Have you saved such gifts — letters, poems or stories? How have those words affected your life? What impact have words had on your illness or tragedy? Our daily lives are often so rushed we don't stop to recognize the positive impact that words have had on us. It sometimes is only after a major illness or another type of tragedy that we take time to evaluate who and what is important to us. We see then that certain people stand out as significant. Think about those who have made a big difference to you. Was it a teacher? A family member? A friend or neighbor? Write about how they influenced or helped you and how your life is richer because of them. The words you write may help take you back to a calmer and more positive time, allowing your mind and body to heal.

Jump Start

When ... said/wrote ... to me, I learned ...

Write about the person's relationship to you and describe what you learned from them.

Tell how their words or actions changed the direction of your life or helped you in some significant way.

Chapter 4

Healing and Feeling

When my mother was diagnosed with lung cancer, I felt at my absolute weakest.

— Jeff Howe

About a half an hour before my next class meeting, I arrived to start setting up tables, chairs, and refreshments. I was eager to begin. I wanted to help students learn to express in writing what we had talked about last time: the fear of dying once we were diagnosed.

Those not dealing with cancer would be given an assignment to write about how and when they learned of the tragedy they were dealing with.

As I looked at the faces of the students coming into the Comedy Theatre, I recognized fear in some of their eyes, uncertainty in others, and a sense of resignation in some of their body language. I know those feelings. Depending on where the patient or caregiver is in the treatment or recovery process, those attitudes change.

Raw fear was what I had experienced that Saturday night years ago.

We were having my teaching colleague and his wife over for dinner.

Bob and I had looked forward to the evening with them and had been preparing for it most of the day. I had waited to take my shower and fix my hair until about 20 minutes before they were due to arrive. I raced to the bathroom, tossed my clothes onto the floor, and jumped into the shower at full speed.

That shower was life changing. Despite being rushed and distracted as I lathered up, I suddenly felt a distinct lump under the skin on my right breast. I immediately stopped, felt it again, and then a shiver went down my spine. It felt like a small marble.

"Not good!" I thought to myself as I felt it again. I had read the articles; I knew this was not normal. I also knew my mammogram six months earlier had shown nothing out of the ordinary.

But I felt even more vulnerable than I would normally. My mother, diagnosed with breast cancer four months earlier, had just undergone a double mastectomy. My brother and I had been told she would not live; it was only a matter of time.

This couldn't be happening.

With a sense of trepidation, I touched the lump again. It was hard and felt flat on one side.

I realized it was almost time for our guests to arrive and knew I had to finish showering and get ready. I didn't mention the lump to Bob.

During dinner, I thought about it several times and knew I would tell him after the guests left.

When I finally told him, I tried to make light of it, something we cancer patients often do when faced with a crisis. It's called denial and some of us are masters at it.

"I found a small lump in my breast while I was showering. I'm sure it's nothing but I'll call the doctor on Monday just to be on the safe side."

He looked worried as we cleaned up the kitchen but told me I was doing the right thing by getting it checked.

A few days later, after seeing my doctor, being referred to a specialist, and undergoing a biopsy on the lump, my surgeon appeared in the outpatient recovery room to talk to me. I was lying on the hospital bed, fearful. I wanted to be hopeful but somehow I knew what the news was going to be. In the operating room I had been awake. Thankfully, my view of the surgery had been blocked by a form draped with hospital-green sheeting.

A local anesthetic was being used. About ten minutes into the surgery, the doctor had suddenly stopped talking. He had been chatting and trying to calm my fears as he was removing the lump, when his mood changed dramatically.

Tension filled the room.

The nurse assisting him squeezed my hand and patted my arm.

When the surgeon told an assistant in the operating room to, "Take the specimen to pathology," he sounded deadly serious.

I was taken to the recovery room. The doctor appeared about half an hour later. As he sat down on my bed, he looked into my eyes and held my hand.

"I was hoping this was not the bad stuff," he said. "But pathology has done a preliminary analysis and, well, it looks like the lump is malignant. I actually saw the blood supply for the tumor when I was operating."

He never used the word cancer. Bad stuff. Tumor. Malignant. Those were the words that echoed through my head.

Fear swept over me. Maybe my mother and I would die together, or perhaps just months apart.

I had a modified radical mastectomy in mid-September. I went to my mother's funeral four weeks later.

So, when I see fear in a cancer patient's eyes, I can relate. When a student enters my class for the first time, we often lock eyes. It's a been-there, done-that moment.

Other people in our families, doctors, or nurses in hospitals give us sympathy or tell us everything will be fine, emphasizing how good we look and how well we are doing. But only another cancer patient can, without saying anything, communicate volumes with a split-second look.

When I first met Joy, I could see she had been through more than I could ever imagine. We didn't lock eyes, though. Joy is blind.

She had heard me give the keynote address on "Silver Saturday" in nearby Pasadena, where breast cancer survivors assembled for seminars and workshops.

Hundreds of women attend the annual gathering, hug one another, and take part in classes on how to deal with the various stages of our disease.

After completing my talk about the positive results participants were experiencing in my Writing for Wellness class, I saw a tall, Black woman in her 50s holding a white cane and being guided by her friend as they approached the podium from the audience.

She seemed burdened with the cares of the world, her shoulders slumped, her face smile-less.

"I need to join your class," she announced in a slight Jamaican accent. "I can't drive and I live in Alhambra (about 15 miles away), but I know I have to be there."

Ellen, her friend, spoke up, "I'll drive you, Joy."

Not only was Joy legally blind, she was also a breast cancer patient and a divorced, single mother with two teenagers. Her mother died of cancer just before Joy was diagnosed, and Joy's husband had left her just prior to that. And I thought I had troubles?

Joy immediately joined my class.

For more than four years, she has managed to get herself to class and back, through the generosity of Ellen and other class members who drive the 30-mile round trip in Los Angeles traffic.

Joy lives on the second floor of a modest apartment building directly beside the San Bernardino Freeway, a major artery into downtown Los

Angeles. An eight-foot cement "sound wall" about 50 feet from her front door thinly masks the vibrations and roar of five lanes of traffic in each direction 24 hours a day. A steep staircase with no landing rises to her doorstep. A sighted person could easily slip and fall. How Joy manages not to is beyond any of those who have ever escorted her home.

She carries a small portable Braille manual typewriter with her and when the class is quiet and students are writing, it clicks and clacks as she takes notes or works on an assignment. Nobody minds the noise.

Joy's poems and prose are often poignant, and as she reads them aloud with eyes closed and head held high, her hands glide across the small Braille dots on her paper. She is an attractive woman with a soothing, almost musical voice.

Healing Words

After discussing their feelings about being diagnosed with cancer or experiencing tragedy, class members spend time writing. Sometimes participants share their work immediately; others choose to wait until the next session to do so after they have time to complete, edit, or rewrite their stories.

As Joy read the words describing her recollections of her diagnosis, the room went silent.

My Season of Grief

The first time I went for a breast biopsy I was told I should come back in six months. It was just a bunch of cysts, the doctor said. No need to operate. Somehow in my spirit I knew it wasn't over, but I was numb and dazed.

And less than a week later I received a telephone call. A team of radiologists had re-evaluated my test and thought I should come back for a biopsy.

The day following the biopsy, I received the diagnosis: cancer.

When my news came, I was already immersed in a season of grief. Because of the recent deaths of my mother and my marriage, I assumed the discovery of the lump in my breast was another harbinger of death, this time my own.

I was already dying emotionally and realized that all I had to do was nothing.

Instead, I chose to fight; there were two children who needed me.

I begged God to just let me live until my daughter turned 18 and then I promised we could renegotiate.

— Joy E. Walker Steward

At age 36, Dave was diagnosed with melanoma. After a course of the drug Interferon failed to stop its spread, Dave tried to qualify for a clinical trial of an experimental drug that might save his life. First, though, he had to qualify, which he equated with trying to obtain a bank loan. As Dave explained, the applicant first has to prove he is solvent enough to repay the loan while also showing he is poor enough to need one. The qualifying tests for the experimental cancer-fighting drugs were similar. Dave's physical condition had to be strong enough for him to endure the treatment, while his cancer had to be aggressive enough to prove he needed it. Almost a Catch-22. He wrote about receiving his results.

Failing the Test

The results of all of my qualifying tests determined: the melanoma had spread to my brain. There were two small tumors caught on a CT scan of my head. They were too small then to cause symptoms, but were definite trouble. The melanoma was continuing to grow in my lungs. I wasn't having trouble breathing yet, but the tumor burden was beginning to get worrisome.

There were undetermined "shadows" in my abdomen. It wasn't clear what the shadows meant, but the news we received already was devastating. The final result was that I did not quality for the clinical trial. We had to deal with these new developments first and fast. I started a leave of absence from work immediately.

— David Key

Jeff, in his late 20s, had recently graduated from college, just gotten married, and was embarking on a promising career as a magazine editor. But the news about his mother's cancer changed everything.

The Emotional Dam

I have always had a scientific mind. While my friends in school feared biology class and cringed at the sight of a Bunsen burner, I was enthralled. So when my mother was diagnosed with lung cancer, I immediately read all about the pathology of the disease, treatment options, and recovery statistics. I wanted to know how much my mom would have to endure — on paper, anyway.

But what it allowed me to do, at least temporarily, was to get lost in the cold scientific minutia of the cancer and to forget for a moment or two that a real person was involved.

Facts don't have feelings; they don't push an agenda. They are what they are, and they leave it up to you to determine whether or not it's good news or bad. When dealing with facts while writing, or even when simply discussing the situation, you can pull away, if only for a few minutes, from the pain that is tugging at you.

While writing, the black and white facts can provide a bridge from one emotion to the next. If healing is achieved through writing, then the writer needs to temper his statements at times with something that is emotionless — the straight facts.

I discovered that if this process isn't adhered to in some way, an emotional dam will break and no one will be able to stick a finger in the holes to keep it from washing away everything.

— Jeff Howe

Lillian was used to helping others. As a licensed vocational nurse, she had cared for many cancer patients throughout her career. It wasn't until her own doctor presented her with bad news that she began to understand how devastating a diagnosis can be.

It's Me and It's Real

A few years back at a regular gynecological visit, my doctor suggested a mammogram, my first. It was a routine procedure and when it came back, he sent me and my x-rays to a surgeon.

I was scared.

The surgeon said I needed a biopsy to see what was really there. Two days later as I came out of the anesthetic, he told me he found a malignancy.

I was shattered to say the least. I was alone, a widow of two years. I asked the doctor what he would suggest if I were his wife.

"I'd want the breast off!" he said.

And, I wanted the same thing. Being a nurse, I had seen a lot and wanted to take no chances.

Two days later, I had a modified radical mastectomy. Something took over and I became a strong, motivated, spiritual being held up by the God I trusted in.

I took my journal with me to the hospital and kept notes of the whole experience.

You would have thought I was at Disneyland. I felt joy and peace. I can't explain it.

A woman who had experienced a mastectomy and was a volunteer came to see me. She was from the American Cancer Society's "Reach for Recovery" group. I asked if I could see her scar. She showed me and answered all my questions.

I know the hardest part for me was looking at my own incisions. Even though I had taken care of patients with the same problem, this was different. This was me and it was real. I felt deformed and like a sideshow freak. I was appalled.

The cancer society had a therapy group for women like myself and it met weekly for 10 or 12 weeks. I decided to attend. It helped so much, so very, very much. We all became friends after the class time was over. Eight or so of us kept meeting and we named ourselves "The Bosom Buddies." We met for a year or two.

I've never had reconstruction. I found no problem wearing a prosthesis.

Two things crucial for me at the time of the crisis in my life were:

1. The writing down of what I was feeling and going through, especially as a fairly new widow and already in a profound grief.

2. Acting on my gynecologist's suggestion that I get a mammogram.

A routine mammogram probably saved my life.

— Lillian M. Pratt, LVN

It's Your Turn

Explain in detail how you found out about an illness or tragedy in your life. Use the exact words you heard. What did the fear feel like? What went through your mind? Try to recapture what you experienced. Recall as many details as you can.

Jump Start

... told me about ... It was (morning, afternoon, evening) when I heard the words ...

I felt ...

After you have written, think about how you felt during and after writing. Did it help you to get out your feelings? What specific emotions resulted?

Part II

Reaching Out, Reaching In

Chapter 5

Thank You

*What do I say to someone who has given me
the gift of life and put the needs of a stranger, my
needs, first?*

— Bill Matteson

Two simple words — thank you — are often the most difficult to say.
When someone compliments an item of our clothing, it is rare for us to
just say, "Thank you."

Much more common is, "Oh, this old thing?" or "I got it on sale."

We sometimes have to practice saying, "Thank you!" Period.

A friend and I have a running joke about this and when one of us
does something nice for the other and the recipient starts to say, "Oh, you
shouldn't have…" the giver of the gift will say, "Read my lips! Thank
you very much."

Thanking a person who has gone above and beyond for you is even
harder. How do you thank a doctor who has saved your life? A simple
thank you doesn't seem enough. You want to pour out your heart in

gratitude but then, when you try, you may feel awkward and end up never thanking them at all.

A bouquet of flowers or a box of candy for a nurse who has seen you through difficult nights is always welcome, but a simple note of thanks may be treasured by that nurse long after the flowers have wilted and the candy has ruined a diet.

Dealing with cancer or other tragedies is difficult for everyone involved. Seeing the fear and pain experienced by many patients causes our closest friends and relatives to recall that they would have gladly changed places with us, taken our burdens away, and undergone the treatments for us, but that was not to be.

Still, those people held our hands, camped out in hospital waiting rooms, drove us to doctors' appointments and treatments, and listened to us when we were angry, sad, or just plain frustrated. We owe them some words of thanks. By writing to them, we, too, will continue to heal.

I remember seeing the sadness in my husband's eyes just before I went into surgery the first time. Clearly, he would have taken my place. He was there for me then and is still here for me every day.

How can I reduce the most important relationship in my life to a few words?

Bob is my husband, my lover, my friend, my personal pilot, and fellow traveler on journeys to Austria's highest mountains and to trails in the bottom of the Grand Canyon. He is my inspiration and the reason behind my academic or career successes.

How do I love him? I can't begin to count the ways. But when I got cancer, he became more than the sum of his parts.

Dear Bob,

Without your help and support during my surgeries, (nine and counting now) I know I wouldn't have gotten well so quickly. You were there to cheer me up when I was blue, hear me out when I was frustrated, and calm me down when every little ache and pain seemed to tell me my cancer was back. You knew just how long to let me wallow and just when to say, "Okay, get in the car; we're going to Starbucks!"

You always made me feel desirable even when I felt ugly and, best of all, you never discounted my feelings when I wanted plastic surgery to make me feel whole again. You assured me that I was fine just as I was and you'd always love me, but if I wanted the surgery you would support that decision, too.

You were my advocate, my advisor, and my rock. Thank you.

I'll love you forever,

Julie

Bob was the first person I saw when I woke up from my first cancer surgery, a mastectomy. I had a hard time with the anesthetic and was ill for many hours afterward. Because of the drugs or my reaction to them, I remember thinking I was being washed down a huge and dark drainpipe. I heard the recovery room nurse saying, "Julie? Don't do that! No! Don't do that!" I guess she didn't want me to go down the drain, either.

I am not a big person and I always wondered if I got the same dose of anesthetics given a 200-pound man. For whatever reason, the whole process wiped me out.

Bob and I had agreed prior to surgery that a "No Visitors" sign on my hospital room would be in order. I had 150 high school students who might want to "visit" me, and the thought, although kind, was just too much. I needed to rest. I also didn't want my students to see me lying in bed in one of those stylish backless gowns with half the ties missing. I didn't even want to think about that scene. No visitors except Bob. Period.

Bob was comforting and reassuring. He told me to rest, and he left the room soon after I woke up and he saw that I was okay. Then I fell back to sleep.

The next thing I knew, one of my high school students who had somehow gotten past the sign was sitting next to my bed holding my hand. I thought I was in some sort of drugged state when I awakened to see him staring at me and looking very sad.

He was 16 at the time and I was his journalism teacher. He liked the subject and he liked me. He was one of my favorite students too, a smart hard-working student who was popular with his peers despite having lots of strong opinions on everything from national politics to vegetarian eating. He recommended drinking sauerkraut juice to everyone.

"You're not going to die are you, Mrs. Davey?" he asked, almost pleading with me.

I was stunned by his question, not one I had been asked before.

"No, Dan, I'm not going to die," I said, genuinely touched by his naïve question and his obvious concern. I tried to muster up a weak smile.

He looked relieved and comforted, and he stood up and left immediately. Clearly, he had received the reassurance he had come for.

Apparently, word had spread through the high school that I had cancer and had been operated on that afternoon. Since Dan did not own a car, he rode his bicycle nearly 10 miles to the Pasadena hospital and sat with tears in his eyes waiting to ask me that question.

After I heard myself reassure Dan that I wasn't going to die, I discovered I had left the realm of self-pity. It was a simple question requiring an equally simple answer. I certainly was not going to die. After all, I couldn't disappoint a 16 year old.

I smile every time I think of his visit. I'm still in touch with Dan Thisdell, who lives in England, is married and the father of three children. We always talk about his hospital visit.

Thanks, Dan, for asking the right question at just the right time.

Many of my students in Writing for Wellness class relate similar stories of friends, family members, and neighbors who help them in various ways while they recover from surgeries, deal with chemotherapy and radiation, or simply provide soft shoulders as needed.

But, when I ask them how many of them have actually written letters or notes of thanks, very few say they have. Some say they have bought and mailed thank you cards with already written verses. No one would be upset to receive one of those. But, how much more personal and touching would a simple heart-felt hand-written note be?

"They took time for us; now we should take time for them," I say to the class members. "But, how do you thank these dear, dear people? Easily, stop thinking about it and, well, just do it."

When these assignments are given in my class, we first discuss who has helped us and who we want to thank. Sometimes it is a doctor, a nurse, or other caregiver in the hospital. Sometimes it is the person nearest and dearest to us.

As some people talk and give examples of those who helped them most, others in the room get ideas and soon everyone is ready to write.

I suggest that participants sit and think about how they felt immediately after receiving the person's help. Reliving those moments provides them with contents for the letters and notes.

Then, and this is essential, I tell them to be very quiet so their words can come out quickly and before they vanish from their minds. Hearing others' voices, music from the radio, or chatter from the television can stop the flow of ideas. Students comment afterwards that these few minutes of quiet are precious to them. We don't often have complete silence in our lives. That alone can be healing.

I usually allow at least 10 minutes of quiet time for people to get started writing down what they have been thinking about. Most have not completely finished in that length of time, but it does allow them to begin.

"Finish that sentence you're writing and in another minute we'll stop. You can continue at home," I tell them.

Then I ask if anyone wants to read what he or she has written. I always stress that this part of class is completely voluntary. I strongly believe that respecting a person's privacy is of utmost importance. Some might feel restricted in their writing if they thought it must be shared later with the group. Students always visibly relax after I explain my "rules."

I am always grateful to students brave enough to share their feelings with others, but I fully understand those who may not feel secure enough to do so. I keep a basket full of "prizes," writing journals and stationery mostly, to award those who take the deep breath and start reading aloud. Sometimes, if someone chokes up while reading, I offer a hug afterward.

In an average college class, only one or two very secure students might take the risk of reading something personal aloud. But in the Writing for Wellness class made up of people who want to write and want to share their feelings, the opposite occurs.

Most people immediately volunteer to read. They seem long past caring about being judged and more concerned about relating to others and learning from them. Refreshing.

The results are excellent because their words and thoughts come straight from their hearts. As they finish reading aloud what they have just written, support for their efforts flourishes as the listeners offer compliments, often mentioning particular excerpts they found especially meaningful. Often times, class members applaud. The enjoyment and fulfillment that readers experience are obvious and an observer can almost see healing begin at those moments.

Healing Words

Sometimes the people you want to thank are the nameless, faceless members of hospital intensive or critical care units, those who kept you alive as you came out of surgery. Or maybe they are the night staff you view merely as silhouettes as they come in from the lighted hallway to take your temperature, check your IV, or put a cool cloth on your forehead. Too ill or too sleepy to completely open your eyes, you often only feel their soft touch or hear their soothing words.

My students agree that a collective thank you is in order from all patients to all such caregivers who spend their nights in ICUs or recovery rooms. Thank you to all of you unheralded angels.

Other individuals, such as those Rick encountered, were almost complete strangers who, it turned out, had more in common with him than anyone could ever imagine. Yet, during his son's illness, Rick had been too wrapped up in his own pain and too concerned with his own son's cancer to properly thank them at the time. But in class, when he read what he wrote to thank two people whose names he never knew, he touched us all.

Midnight Vigil

Their son was dying; maybe mine was, too. While I was unsure, they were not.

It was just about midnight as I was leaving the Bone Marrow Transplant (BMT) unit at City of Hope, when I exchanged a greeting with a couple, also on their way out.

They asked how my son was doing. Perhaps they'd seen me there before. I was vaguely aware that they had been visiting their son, whom I thought later may have been the patient bound in gauze, full-body gauze, in the room two doors down from my son's.

Those days I had a perpetual catch in my throat, which intensified before each visit to my son Rick, 37, who had just undergone a bone marrow transplant.

I seemed to be joined emotionally with each support person I saw, whether we spoke or not, whether our eyes met or not.

That night I told the couple that Rick was okay so far, but not yet out of the woods.

They smiled and wished me well. We went to our separate cars.

I never asked them about their own son who I learned died the next day. Looking back, I wish that I'd had their acceptance, their strength. They seemed at peace. I wasn't.

I wish that I'd known their son was the one in jeopardy.

They took time to ask about my son while theirs was dying. I have not forgotten that encounter, perhaps because of guilt.

I had, after all, failed to thank them or to ask about him, maybe because they were together, coping with the worst loss a parent can suffer.

Yet they had paused that fatal night to ask me how things were going.

In our labors, it was they who felt sympathy for me.

Their vigil was over.

Mine continued.

— Rick Myers

At the Mayo Clinic, Charles had undergone a series of medical tests, all of which he flunked, and he was being pushed in a wheelchair by a staff member back to the waiting area.

As they turned the corner, Charles saw his wife Elena standing there exclaimed to the staff member, "How beautiful a sight!"

Elena was there for him despite his condition, his test results, and what the future might hold.

Back at their home in Hawaii, Charles composed the following using his exclamation as its title.

How Beautiful a Sight

A morning's chill before first sight
Wakes me before first light
And I seem as in a vague dream;
Then morning's sounds intervene;
A gecko who resides with us
Calls to someone repeatedly;
The ceiling fan keeps its pulse rhythmically;
And at first light the birds declare their plight,
Or perhaps they speak of other things;
After a while, at first sight,
I see you lying there, asleep,
Your face beautiful
But your hair in disarray.
I wouldn't have it any other way.
How beautiful a sight
To see at first light
The woman who has loved and cared for me,
And whom I love wholeheartedly!

— Charles F. Fell

Dave was in the midst of the fight for his life when he published a thank you article about his wife, Janis, his caregiver. She was surprised and overwhelmed by his words. To update them on his condition, Dave had developed a newsletter titled DO-IT, (Dave's Own Inspirational Team), which he sent to friends and family members. Janis cherishes this gift of words.

Angel at My Bedside

I would like to give tribute to Janis, my wife, who has endured this entire cancer saga alongside me. She has been with me during every doctor's appointment, X-ray, CAT scan, blood test, radiation treatment, chemotherapy, Interleukin-2 hospitalization, and surgery.

She has seen to it that I'm as comfortable as I can be, given the circumstances.

She has sacrificed her career goals to be at my bedside in the hospital and to care for me at home. Her dedication to the mission of my being cancer-free is absolutely complete.

To understand the scope of this effort, one must realize that this has been going on every day, seven days a week, month after month, for over two years. She is there to hold me up while I vomit, provide a cold washcloth when I'm feverish, draw up the blankets when I'm shivering, make me feel secure during my hallucinations, and bring me my medications with a smile. She cleans my atrial catheter at home, never once missing the daily flushing.

She maintains the household, including juggling the bills, seeing that the house is kept up and the animals are fed and that someone will come to feed them while we are on one of our many trips to the hospital.

She encourages me when I'm down, lets me cry when I need to, and sometimes cries alongside me. She helps keep in touch with my family, especially the kids. In short, she sees that our lives continue to function through all the disruptive clutter of undergoing cancer treatments.

She is truly the angel at my bedside.

I dedicate this month's newsletter to Janis. She has demonstrated both her commitment to fighting cancer and her unyielding love for me.

I pledge my unending love to her.

— David Key

Donna's cancer had returned several times. She knew her support network helped her battle the disease and she wrote the following to thank them.

Branches of a Mighty Oak

Four years have passed since I was first diagnosed with breast cancer at age 36. From day one I had a positive, fighting spirit.

My plan:

I would bravely endure all necessary treatments and side effects.

I would gain courage from the Bible and from cancer survivors' success stories.

I would tackle whatever came my way in order to get this behind me, so that I could move on with my normal life of teaching, carpooling my three kids to their activities, and supporting my husband.

Well, here we are four years later. My cancer has returned several times. It is now in my lung and bones, but guess what? My plan remains the same. Endure, gain strength from others' successes, and tackle what comes my way. My husband says, "These are the cards we were dealt, and we will deal with them." One day at a time we deal with it.

At the time I laid out my plan, I left out one important component — support. In my battle, support from others ended up being one of the major factors in my day-to-day successes. Your supporters can be an organized group, co-workers, neighbors, family and friends, a counselor, a religious institution, a hospital, etc.

In the beginning, I didn't see that receiving support from others was going to affect how my journey with cancer would play out. Now I get it and it's HUGE! Your supporters help you find joy in life. They lift you up when you don't even know you need lifting. They are there with you when you are awake in the middle of the night even though you don't see them. You feel their love long after they have left your presence.

My support system is like a huge oak tree. Its branches keep extending and extending, sometimes overlapping. So I would now like to adjust my "plan" to include:

Seek support from others. Embrace others' support and let it carry me.

Thank you to everyone in my life who has come forward to support me in this challenging time. You carry me day to day.

With love,

Donna

— Donna Logan

Marilyn wanted to thank her daughter but couldn't seem to find the right words until she came to Writing for Wellness class and was given an assignment to write someone a thank you note. She wrote a note and a poem to honor her daughter.

My Daughter, My Friend

When I think of you, I think of the beauty that you are and the beauty that is in you. I think of the joy I feel in your presence, the joy of having you come and go in my daily life. I think of our laughing together and sharing the same sense of humor. I think of how we work and play and live so comfortably together. When I think of you, I think of gratitude, a gratitude that I've always felt having you as my daughter, and now, since cancer so inconveniently entered my life, I think of you with a gratitude that is too deep to express.

You have been my rock of support.

You have been my personal angel.

You have walked the walk with me every step of the way

Through discovery and doctor visits
Through diagnosis and surgery
Through chemotherapy and radiation
Through infusions and endless labs
Through shots and drains and nausea
Through weight loss and weakness
Through every hair that fell
Through every funny scarf and hat and wig
That covered, as you called it,
Your "mom's cute little, bald head."
Through hair growing back
Through strength returning
Through all the ups and all the downs
You were there
for me
by me
with me.
Because of you, I was not alone,
and that made all the difference.
Thank you, my Daughter, my Friend.

— Marilyn Butler

Christine, early 30s, waiting for her first bone marrow transplant, shares the fear and frustrations she feels the night before her surgery to insert a Hickman catheter into a major artery. In her journal, she thanks Sean, a fellow cancer patient in his 20s, for providing the strength she needed.

Badge of Honor

I'm scared. So many friends and I don't know who to talk to. The truth is, not everyone is good to talk to. The truth is, I'm not usually better off after talking to someone. The people I want to reach for are other cancer patients.

Besides my parents, Sean is the only person I had the energy to talk to tonight. He's another young cancer patient. He immediately put me at ease and made me not so scared. He put strength back into my spine.

When I whined about getting a Hickman catheter in my chest and worried about the scar it would leave, he told me, "This is war! The Hickman will save your veins. Wear it as a badge of honor!"

He told me the bone marrow transplant would be the most awesome thing that would ever happen to me because it would save my life.

He made me feel thankful instead of spiteful.

Thank you, Sean.

This is why "normal healthy people" no matter how well-meaning, cannot help as much as people who have actually gone through cancer. Normal people just don't have the perspective of experience. Normal people don't usually face their own mortality on a daily basis.

We cancer patients have no other choice.

— **Christine Pechera**

It's Your Turn

I always remind my students that everyone has written a thank you note in his or her lifetime. Our parents told us it was the right thing to do. It still is. The stationery isn't important; the words are.

Be as specific as you can to make the note personal. Go beyond saying, "I don't know what I would have done without you." Explain why, "Having you take care of the kids has meant everything to me because I can concentrate on getting well, knowing they are in your hands."

A thank you note is usually short, to the point, and fairly easy to do. Once it has been written and delivered, we feel a sense of relief and peace. You know people in your life who deserve your thanks. Use your own words or use those below to help you get started.

Journalists often begin articles using the person's name.

Jump Start

Dear ...:

Without your help I ...

This is a simple way to begin. There are thousands of other ways. What is important is to relate to another person in your own words. Imagine receiving such a note or letter from a friend or loved one. Would you be concerned with spelling, handwriting, or punctuation? No. You would be overwhelmed that the person took time to put his or her feelings into words.

What could be more important to the sender? What could be more precious for the recipient? After you have finished writing, see how you feel. If you feel better, perhaps you have just discovered a new form of "therapy." I always stress to the class that, when appropriate, the writer should take the next step and mail or deliver the letter or note to the person who helped them. Or, if the person is in another state, read the note over the phone before mailing it.

Many times the writer wants to recopy the letter onto nice stationery or check the spelling. Whatever makes you comfortable should be done. Timing is important for giving the person your note, too. Some wait for a quiet evening; others want the whole family to be present when it is read aloud.

Chapter 6

Love Letters

Love, like water, must move or else it will stagnate.
It must flow. It can heal. It can cleanse.
But, if not cared for, it will evaporate.
We are conduits for this great force.
— Christine Pechera

When you think of love letters, you might imagine those personal, often mushy ones that lovers write to one another, the ones tied up with pastel ribbons, sprinkled with perfume, and hidden away on a closet shelf.

But I ask my Writing for Wellness class to write another kind of love letter — one to someone they miss, someone who they love dearly and who has significantly changed their lives. The person may or may not still be alive.

Because I have personally experienced cancer twice, and have also dealt with it on many other levels, having lost both my parents (Edward Lynn and Mozelle), my sister-in-law (Jan), my college roommate (Mary), an especially close girlfriend (Josephine), a cousin (Ruby Jo), and the husbands of three dear friends (Bill, Esker, and Jim), I feel I can help others deal with tragedies in their own lives.

Over the 18 years I taught college writing, I found students frequently had confided in me and had also written about the illnesses and tragedies of their friends, parents, and spouses.

I give a regular assignment called "Missing Persons" in which students often write about those they have lost contact with or others from whom they have separated. But, each semester, a few of the students also write about major losses in their lives — a son or daughter taken in illness or in an accident, a parent who died without warning, or a friend who died of a drug overdose.

One night in my college writing class when students brought in their assignments from the week before, I asked if anyone would volunteer to share what they wrote about a "Missing Person" in their lives.

Several of the 19-year-olds wrote about a favorite cousin their age who had moved away or a grandmother or grandfather in another state. Their pieces were full of nostalgia. We smiled. Everyone felt good.

Then one student, a 40-year-old deputy sheriff, tall and powerful looking in his 200-pound frame, raised his hand. He was dressed in his uniform, which added to the aura of strength he projected. I expected a police story of some sort, perhaps about another officer, a partner, who had been transferred.

But when he began to read about his father's death, the mood in the classroom became one of stunned silence. Everyone looked first at him, then at me.

He read only two lines and then couldn't continue. His eyes flooded with tears and he choked up. He handed his paper to me and gestured for me to continue reading aloud. Clearly he wanted to share what he had written. It was poignant and full of the love a son had for a father missing in his life. Tears rolled down both of his cheeks the entire time I read his words.

After class, the deputy thanked me for providing the opportunity for him to deal with his grief. His father had died several years before, but the seemingly tough officer had never completely accepted the loss or written about it until that evening. He said he felt much better having expressed his feelings and he hoped to continue the process as he faced other tragedies in his personal life and in his career as a law enforcement officer.

So, when I ask Writing for Wellness students to write about "Missing Persons," I know it might bring tears as they remember someone who has passed away, but I also feel it can be a prescription for healing.

For those in the class who may not have taken the time to express how much they love someone and then find it is too late, it could also be a chance to say goodbye.

As the pieces are read aloud, we learn that some of their loved ones have died peacefully in their sleep; others have been victims of tragic accidents.

There is one common thread. All are missed by their survivors.

Healing Words

When Yuan Mao Xie, 40, first joined Writing for Wellness class she told the group that she was there mainly to learn to improve her English. She may not have fully understood that the class was one aimed at writing to heal.

Yuan, in her lab coat, came to class on her lunch hour.

A cancer research associate at City of Hope, she, along with hundreds of others, is searching for a cure for cancer.

An immigrant from mainland China, she spoke with a strong accent and was very shy, looking down at her paper whenever she read. Her voice was whisper soft and her words almost apologetic. Over the months, her shyness disappeared and she began to write more openly about the tragedies in her own life, tragedies she had not brought up when first-day introductions were made.

We learned that her father, Mao Hai Kun had died in China of brain cancer at age 70, while Yuan was living in the United States. Due to political restrictions, she was not able to re-enter China to attend her father's funeral and had continued to mourn him.

Here is her letter, read through her tears.

Dear Father,

I miss you very much, especially when I am having fun playing with my kids or when I am relaxing at home. I want to tell you that I am doing well. I have a happy family and am doing research to fight cancer.

My husband, You Qin, and I have two lovely children, Jamie and Jason.

Jamie, seven years old, is a top student in her class and loves drawing and playing the piano. She is talented in both.

Jason, three years old, is an active, smart boy and a handsome boy.

I have taught them how to say grandpa in Chinese and I showed them a picture of you and told them, "Grandpa is in heaven now and loves you very much."

— Yuan Mao Xie

One assignment I give is for students to explain what the Dickens' quote from A Tale of Two Cities, *"It was the best of times; it was the worst of times" means in their own lives.*

As Annie read her love letter, everyone wiped tears from their eyes.

Dearest Brad,

The best part of your cancer was my finding you. The worst part of your cancer was my losing you. We had barely a year together, but I hold each memory in my heart like stardust in a locket. I've gone over and over in my mind so many times, asking why God brought us together.

I remember one thing that your mother said. She had always wondered why her son had never married by the age of thirty-five, such a good-looking young man with such charm. She said it must have been because he had been waiting for me. We were meant to have that last year of your life together.

As your mother once told me, "Brad helped you to live again and you helped him to die."

Always and Forever, Annie.

— Annie Watson

The night before her first bone marrow transplant Christine wrote a letter to her younger brother, Francis Rex, who had died of cancer at age 16. He had also gone through a bone marrow transplant 15 years earlier, but died two years later. Christine had been the donor for Rex's transplant.

Dear Rex,

Wherever you may be, you are always with me. I ask for your help and strength through this. I know it must be a walk in the park compared to what you went through. You were so young, but you were not frightened.

You may have been scared from time to time, but you never complained. People may say I am an inspiration, but I am a fraud compared to you.

You were the true hero and warrior. Why do the good die young? I wish I could have shared more of this life with you. May God bless you always. You will always be in my heart. Tonight, somehow I know I am not alone.

Love, Christine

— Christine Pechera

Losing any loved one is painful; losing your child is unthinkable. The continuing and quiet anguish that parents, parents of any age, go through is difficult to imagine. Many express their feelings years, even decades later. Others never do.

Tony Garcia, 47, attended one of the first classes of Writing for Wellness. His wife, Bonna, works at City of Hope and had seen the flyer announcing the time and place. When he entered the room, he seemed uncomfortable at first, as if he did not quite know why he had come.

But when introductions were made, Tony revealed that his 27-year-old son, Casey, had been killed in a car accident. When he read his letter at the next class meeting, we all shed tears for a young man we never knew and for his father who we could see had suffered greatly.

Here is part of Tony's letter to Casey.

Dear Casey,

When I think of the time you and I spent together camping in the Sierras, fishing our hearts out, just the two of us, it takes me back to your childhood when I first introduced you to my favorite pastime. You were only about four years old at the time, and the idea of standing in the same place for hours on end, waiting for a fish to come by and tug on your line seemed to be more than you could tolerate. But when one finally did, your eyes would light up, and you would become so excited, you could hardly control yourself. As the years went by, your fishing skills improved to the point where you were always out-fishing me.

Your love for the outdoors was obvious, so I took you fishing as often as I could. As you approached your early teens, you became interested in other things. You bought your first car with money that you had saved from your after school job at McDonald's, a 1978 Toyota that needed a paint job and new upholstery, but you were pretty proud of it just the same.

You were always improving it, putting other little touches on it that made it unique. And when your friends saw what you had done to your car, they soon copied your style. So you would change it again, make it unique to fit your personality. You always stayed a step or two ahead of the game when it came to your cars. I'm sure you didn't realize it at the time, but they were playing follow the leader, and you were in front.

As you grew older, the fishing trips became a little less frequent, but you and I still went to the Sierras a couple times a year, and you continued to out-fish me. You became the teacher, and I became the student.

Your cars evolved to newer, fancier, shinier ones that went faster and faster. Your mom was always afraid you were going to kill yourself or someone else with those little "pocket rockets" (as you liked to call them), but you were always careful, never reckless. We were so thankful when you decided to trade the fast little car in on a new four-wheel-drive truck. Little did we know you would start customizing the truck right after you bought it.

Everything you did, you put your heart into, made sure it was done right, or you would do it over and over again, until it was as close to perfect as you could get it.

I don't think I told you often enough, son, but you made mom and me so proud, because with you, good enough was never good enough. You never did anything half way. You always put 100% of your effort into everything you did. You were the best son that anybody could ever ask for, Casey.

Your mom and I knew you were special, but we never imagined just how special you would be. When you married a girl who had a child from someone else, and we saw just how much you loved that little boy, as if he were your own, we knew you were going to be the best father a kid could have.

How sad that just eleven days after you were married, you would be taken from us by a senseless act of carelessness by someone who had no business being behind the wheel of a moving vehicle. Our lives are shattered; our hearts are broken. And not a day, or even a minute goes by that your mom and I don't think of you.

We miss you so much, your beautiful face, the way you used to hug us, the sound of your voice.

I lie awake at night, watching the bedroom door, expecting to see you at any moment, walking down the hall, saying, "night mom; night pop" the way you used to do.

I can no longer bring myself to go fishing in the Sierras, or anywhere else for that matter. It just isn't the same anymore.

I would gladly give up my life if I could have just one more fishing trip with you, even if for just a few hours. It would mean so much to your mom and me to tell you just one more time, to your face, how much we love you.

I miss you, son. I miss you every day, every hour, every minute. The pain and emptiness your mom and I feel is unbearable at times. We feel as if we have lost everything, because to us, you were everything.

For everyone around us, our family, our friends, our co-workers, life has gone back to normal. When we are with them, we try to act as normal as we can, but your mom and I will never feel "normal" again.

We look at your pictures every day. We look forward to the day we are all together again. Until that day comes, my son, know that we love you, and that you are with us in our hearts always.

With all my love, Dad.

— Tony Garcia

It's Your Turn

Write a letter to someone missing in your life. Write about the good times you shared and describe why you miss them today. What humorous parts of your life do you remember sharing with them? What did they help you through? When do you miss them most — holidays, quiet times, sports events, hearing music you both loved?

Jump Start

The first two or three words you use in a letter will help you get started.

Christmas wasn't the same this year without you because ...

Raising two children alone has been ...

Today would have been our/your (anniversary, special event we celebrated, favorite meal, or family holiday) ...

Share your letter with a person who knew or was related to your loved one or friend. Your words may help you remember the good times. Your letter is a tribute, too, to the memory of someone who made a significant difference in your life.

Chapter 7

Private Anguish

Where's God?
Damn it! I can't find God!
I pray. It's empty!

— Theda Clark

Suffer in silence. Some of us do that. Others are the screamers, whiners, let-it-all-out types. Sometimes they have it easier. Everyone knows when they are frightened, angry, frustrated. People around them try to comfort them and cheer them up. And sometimes that seems to work.

Other people smile, put on a good front, and reassure their families and friends. No one can even imagine what is going on inside of them. Expressing sadness, fear, and frustration is difficult. Some say it is even more difficult than dealing with the disease or tragedy itself.

"I can handle the chemo and radiation," one student said in class. "It's the fear and sadness that consume me."

Our friends and family members know that physical healing is a

69

process that takes time. We have an operation or a procedure; we slowly get better. People expect that and have a certain amount of tolerance for it. But often those around us may expect us to "get over it" psychologically more quickly than we might be able to. We might even expect ourselves to recover sooner than we can.

My cancer operation was not all that painful, physically. I remember taking some pain medications in the hospital and then only using Tylenol or aspirin when I got home. I was back teaching my high school classes in four weeks. That was the easy part.

I had chosen the modified mastectomy rather than the lumpectomy, having talked with my doctors who recommended it as more of a sure thing, a good way to ensure they got all the cancer. Nancy Reagan, with all her fame and money, had the same operation. Before her, Betty Ford and Happy Rockefeller, again, very wealthy women with top medical advisors had also taken that path.

I felt I had made the right decision. Still, there was that scar, that flatness, that feeling of being lopsided. I found myself resigned to it and felt I was recovering both physically and psychologically. Bob helped a great deal and told me from his heart that he loved me even more than before, having almost lost me. I remember him saying, "If you have to have cancer, breast cancer is probably the one to have. At least there's an accepted treatment with a good chance for success."

I knew he was right. It was logical. I felt better, reassured. For a while.

A few weeks following my surgery, I was fitted with a prosthesis and I felt good just to be doing routine things — going to the market or filling up the car. I thought I was healed and back to normal. I wasn't.

It was one Sunday morning when a family member from out of state called to ask how I was doing. We chatted a while and she seemed genuinely concerned about my well-being. Then, out of nowhere it seemed, she asked why I had made the choice to have the mastectomy. I was shocked by her words and her almost arrogant tone.

"I just can't believe you chose to be disfigured like that. I've read articles that say having the lumpectomy is just as safe. Why would you do that?"

She continued to talk but I didn't hear anything else she said.

Disfigured! Disfigured! The word cut more deeply than the surgeon's knife. Is that how the world would view me?

Immediately following my surgery, I had felt relieved to be rid of the cancer. I didn't even need chemotherapy because the tumor was contained and had not spread to my lymph nodes. The doctors assured me that I was one of the lucky ones. But, following that conversation, I was devastated.

I had a hard time shopping for clothes. Even seeing low-cut dresses or tight-fitting sweaters on mannequins in store windows left me depressed. I avoided going into department stores.

I felt angry at my situation and frustrated that I had cancer while so many other women did not. I knew it was a juvenile attitude; I couldn't help it. I stopped buying anything but loose-fitting clothing. I found myself wearing layers, suits, jackets — covering myself up. When I wasn't at work, I wore sweat suits. I was grateful to be cancer-free, but I didn't feel normal.

I had always loved swimming. How could I swim with a rubbery, floppy prosthesis? What if it floated away in the pool?

Then, I decided to try to adjust to my plight. I bought a "mastectomy" swimsuit, one with a cloth pocket to hold the prosthesis in place, joined the YMCA and enrolled in water aerobics classes. Still, I felt odd and I often changed clothes in the toilet stall, not out in the locker room with all the other naked ladies.

It wasn't until I had to have a second mastectomy 14 years later and underwent what my plastic surgeon at the time, Dr. Gordon Sasaki, called "restorative" surgery that I felt almost normal again. He told me he thought the term "reconstruction" was best used to describe rebuilding collapsed structures, not bodies. He knew I taught English and thought I might appreciate the explanation. I agreed completely. We both got a laugh out of it.

At Dr. Sasaki's suggestion, I got breast implants. Heck, we were only a few miles from Hollywood; I would be as "normal" as hundreds of other women on Sunset Boulevard. But, it wasn't an overnight process. I first had tissue expanders implanted to allow skin to stretch and grow so it would cover the implants. Today, I understand, this is done at the same time as the mastectomies. It took several months before I had grown enough of my own tissue to cover the implants that were to be placed during a five-hour surgery.

I recovered quickly and I was happy. I could buy fitted dresses, regular swimsuits and even wear sweaters. My period of private misery was over. At least I thought so then.

My reactions seem to be common among those who suffer in silence. Beating cancer isn't the whole battle. Ultimately, we must feel comfortable with what remains of us physically and psychologically.

Healing Words

Our individual stories of what causes our private anguish are unique. Some people have strong support systems as friends and family rally to their bedsides. But, even for them, it may be the ravages of chemotherapy or radiation that cause depression.

Others have relatively little physical reaction to the chemotherapy or radiation, yet they feel desperately lonely and isolated. Surprisingly, over the more than five years of classes, several participants in Writing for Wellness have revealed that once they were diagnosed, their partners, spouses, or roommates found their situations too stressful and left, moved out, or divorced them. The patients all admitted that their relationships were already in trouble prior to the life-threatening illnesses or other tragedies. That was merely the straw that broke the camel's back. Still, they were left alone.

Here are expressions of anguish written by students in my class — a patient, a wife, a daughter, a son, and a friend.

Doug, 37, had just ended a long-term relationship when he was diagnosed with B-cell, diffuse, non-Hodgkin's lymphoma. He was desperately ill, could not work, and needed an autologous (his own) stem cell transplant to survive. Doug not only had to deal with his illness, but also with his lost love. His poems reflect his anguish.

Dead Ringer

I listen
to the phone
not ringing
and I know
it's you
not calling me.

— Doug Wilkey

Never

If you were here
could I deceive you?
or could you convince me
all was okay,
or just go away?

Never knew you'd
never stay.
Never heard what you'd
never say.

— Doug Wilkey

Edna's mother had hidden her own anguish, and her daughter followed her mother's example.

Silent Burdens

When I was 21 years old my mother died of leukemia. It was a slow and painful death, and it changed me forever. We were very close, as close as mother and daughter could be.

In her attempt to protect me and my sister from the truth of her condition, my mother had decided that she should shield us from many of the details surrounding her disease. In fact, we never heard the word "leukemia" mentioned. We were only told she had "a problem with her blood."

I saw her descend from a smart, active, vibrant woman, and a lover of life, to someone who could not get out of bed due to her anemia and pain. She never complained during those two years, and it wasn't until a week before her death that I learned the truth about the nature of her illness, and that it was terminal.

After she died, my world fell apart. I was consumed with a grief so powerful that, after a few weeks of it, my mind could not handle what had happened and blissfully sent me into a numbed state that lasted for months. I say "blissfully," but in reality I was like the undead, going about my business and trying to be normal, but feeling nothing, neither happiness nor sadness. Just numb. Frozen.

It seemed obscene to me that other people were enjoying their lives, or at least getting through them without the pain I was experiencing. Didn't they realize my mother had died? How could everyone behave as if nothing had happened?

My mother died during the summer between my junior and senior years at UCLA. When I returned to school in September, I met up with an acquaintance from my art history classes. She asked how my summer had been.

"Fine," I replied.

I could not permit myself to confide in anyone, because I was afraid of the emotions that might spill out.

— Edna Teller

Janis and David Key were married two years after he was diagnosed with melanoma at the age of 35. He died one year and three days after their wedding day. She was his caregiver, an often exhausting and forgotten role filled by spouses, friends, and family members in hospitals and homes throughout the country while all of the attention goes to the patient. Caring for the caregiver is sometimes not even in the picture.

Overlooked and Under-appreciated

Being a caregiver of a loved one with cancer can be a thankless, and at times, very lonely job. I have always been a strong and capable woman whose second nature is to nurture and care for others.

At the time Dave had been battling cancer for more than two years. Although I would never wish cancer on anyone, Dave benefited from being the victim, quickly establishing a support team to encourage and help him, while I steadfastly sat on the sidelines cheering him on, but garnering little attention or support for myself.

I don't want to sound like one who is full of self-pity, but dealing with cancer took its toll on me as well.

As his IL-2 treatment approached, my own anxiety mounted, knowing the seriousness of the procedure and facing the real possibility he might die. However, when I tried to share my concerns and feelings with Dave, he was unable to help. Rightfully so, he was overwhelmed with his own anxieties, but we were husband and wife and I needed him, too.

As our tensions increased, we finally came to a crisis point and engaged in verbal sparring. Through the anger, something I said must have stuck with him and gave him pause to consider my situation. After he recovered from that treatment, he wrote his tribute to me (see p. 54).

Prior to it, Dave had never mentioned my struggle, but from then on, he made sure he included me in his unfolding story.

As the song goes, "You always hurt the one you love." I definitely felt taken for granted at times during our battle against cancer. Dave loved me with his heart and soul and I loved him just as much. I know he never meant to hurt me, but he trusted in our love to weather any storm, sometimes without considering the impact on me.

— Janis Garrett

Jeff writes openly about his first thoughts after hearing the news about his mother's cancer.

Mirror, Mirror

I hate looking in the mirror. Not because my hair won't sit straight or a pimple just had to announce itself on the tip of my nose, but because of what I see inside. I think everyone has this concern; I haven't met a person yet who is completely happy with his or her inner self.

For me, though, I think I'm a pretty good, stable person (though I am married, and you know what in-laws can do to your stress level). But the ill will I harbor toward my reflection became painfully noticeable after my mother was diagnosed with lung cancer.

Suddenly, I thought about myself more than I ever had. How would her situation change my life? What responsibilities would I have to shoulder? Would my wife and I still be able to move out of state?

These were legitimate questions, I'm sure, but what shook me was that they were some of the first questions to reach my conscious mind.

Forget that my mother could die soon and that my father would have his world and everything he ever knew snatched from him. This was about my life, dammit, and this wasn't fair! Well, no dude, it ain't.

Despite the formation of logical, cogent thoughts about how the disease affected my family, I couldn't get my head around the fact that I was being a Grade-A jerk about this, and it really upset me.

I had always been the strong one, the rock to whom everyone else could anchor and ride out whatever storm was brewing. But when I looked around, seeking a safe harbor for myself, I didn't know where to go. But I did know that someone had to smack me around a little!

I didn't like the fact that I spent so much time worrying about how my life would change because of my mother's cancer. I was in my 20s, and I certainly didn't want to have a dependent pushing 60!

Why, oh why, couldn't my heart make my head understand that it was exactly what I should have been thinking about? I had people who needed me, and my own petty problems were not an issue. I had one parent who was sick, and I had another with a sick heart.

I should have worried about the wonderful woman who was destined to a difficult remainder of her life, or about an incredible man who sometimes needs a shoulder to lean on.

I should have worried about a family unit that may someday soon need another rope to hold it together, and that might be me.

So, I took another look in the mirror and I realized that as much as I purported to be a giving, helpful person, I was an incredibly selfish one. My mother's cancer wasn't about me. It was never about me, and will never be about me. It is about her and what she needs. And if I can reconcile that, if I can recognize that, then I will be able to be there when she needs me.

— Jeff Howe

Close friends of cancer patients also suffer along with family members, sometimes carrying unspoken burdens. Kathryn, a writer (Author of Music as a Healing Tool*), a singer, an actress, and an assistant pastor in the Lutheran Church, has been Linda Bergman's dear friend for more than 25 years. In some cases, friends such as Kathryn and Linda grow even closer than sisters as they face adversity together. Kathryn writes about how Linda's cancer taught her the meaning of unconditional love.*

Soul Mates

In an age when we tend to throw around terms like "unconditional love" with seeming earnestness and ease, I don't feel we can ever really know what that term means until we've been truly challenged with a serious illness of the person who is the object of our declared devotion.

Finding out that my best friend, Linda, on her 50th birthday, had received the horrible news of her leukemia diagnosis was too much to bear. I simply could not process it. She had been through so much already. Her prior health setbacks were difficult, frightening, and frustrating for her and everyone concerned.

For me, it was never an issue or an inconvenience to be there for her during the years of various health crises. She was my beloved friend.

"Unconditional love" was at the core of our friendship. Embracing her new leukemia status became my reality now, not theories or fluffy adages. I experienced the normal, clichéd feelings: she was simply too young for this, and it just wasn't fair. But deep inside, I knew that trying to keep her spirits up through positive energy, prayers, love, and humor was essential.

This was all based on the Linda I had known from the start and the friendship we had cultivated and trusted.

To me, our kind of extraordinary friendship had been like a marriage, "'til death do us part" being central to our sacred oath. But, the true test is how we choose to react in times of trial.

Do I succumb to my own fears, lack of control, and impatience, or do I get off myself and meet each challenge of her illness by asking myself, "Is my love for my friend stronger than, larger than, my own fears?"

Of course.

Then I could proceed from strength, helping rather than hindering her day.

To see Linda, my astonishingly gifted, intelligent, loving, feisty Irish friend, reduced to trying to contact her husband Chuck by using her television remote control, instead of her cell phone, was one of countless emotionally challenging moments during her illness and treatment phase.

But reacting with grace or humor always remained so much larger than my fears. Focusing on who she really was, not who she became during the ravages and alterations of her medications made it easier to help her get back to herself.

Unconditional love is indeed possible.

— Kathryn Skatula

Jerome, 40s, father of two, is an actor and a filmmaker. He is also a cancer patient in immediate need of a bone marrow transplant. If he does not find a donor, he will die. Because of his mixed-race background, it has been impossible at this writing to find a donor match for him. He is a man of faith and he is holding out hope, but in his private moments, he thinks ahead to his children's futures and hopes he will be there to share memories with them.

Why Am I This Way?

I've been described as heroic, energetic, enthusiastic, kind-hearted, a positive life force, and an example for others, and a pleasure to have around. I've also been described as a dear friend and an inspiration. And then, there's that time when someone mentioned that a mutual friend thought that I was in denial.

On February 11, 2003, I was diagnosed with chronic myeloid leukemia or CML. I've been told that I'm in critical need of a marrow donor and my time is running out. Friends, family, and those that know of my story often wonder why I don't spend my days dwelling on this illness. In fact, I rarely think about it, not because I'm in denial, but because I choose not to let it overtake my life. Quite frankly, I'm too busy saving lives (as I see it) by educating and registering minorities to become marrow donors.

Maybe that's why I identify with the comic book character Superman. Seriously, as long as I don't dwell on how life would be for my two children if I were not here for them, I can go forward and do what needs to be done. As Morgan Freeman once said in a movie, "You either have to get busy living or get busy dying."

Why am I this way? That's a more difficult question to answer. What I do know for sure is that I'm the proud father of Cameron, 16, and

Mikayla, 12. Cameron, my son, is one of the most honest, good-hearted, and smartest young men that I know. And he plays a mean viola! Mikayla has a warm heart, is smart, beautiful, and a talented ballerina.

My children are my inspiration and I want them to know that life is worth fighting for. And the best way for me to do that is to fight this battle for myself, for others in my predicament, and especially for them. Truthfully, I can't see myself wasting time worrying about something that only God and my faith in Him can cure.

Do not misunderstand; I have my moments of despair. Writing about this now is difficult to do, not because I'm afraid of dying but because I'm afraid of not being here to watch my children have children of their own, grandchildren I can help raise and spoil every chance I get.

So why am I this way?

I'm this way because this is the way God made me.

I will end with one of my favorite sayings, "God is good; His mercy is everlasting; and His truth endures through all generations."

— Jerome G. Williams

It's Your Turn

Are you faking a strong front by putting on a happy face for those around you? Are your own fears keeping you from helping a friend or family member with cancer? How do you really feel about what you are going through? Does anyone know? Expressing your fears and frustrations might help you heal. Writing may help chase some of the demons from your mind and body. Think about what Doug, Edna, Janis, Jeff, Kathryn, and Jerome have revealed. Are you able to talk about your feelings with anyone?

Start to write about the facts and feelings of your experience.

Jump Start

A journalist might ask you to explain facts and feelings of your situation with questions based on the following:

What hurt me most was when ...

I have a hard time telling anyone about ... because ...

I am disappointed/shocked at my reaction about ... because ...

I learned about what really matters in life when ...

Note how you feel after writing. Perhaps you will be confident enough to share what you have gone through by talking to a friend or family member about it or by sharing what you have written.

Chapter 8

Changing Priorities

For everyone around us, life has gone back to normal. When we are with them, we try to act normal, but your mom and I will never feel "normal" again.

— Tony Garcia

I call them impatient patients. Isn't that an oxymoron? Whatever its title, I have experienced in myself and witnessed in others an actual syndrome that nearly all of us have exhibited at one time or another and to one degree or another.

The scenario:

You have been told you have a serious illness or someone in your family has been involved in a tragedy. After the initial shock, something happens. The everyday "problems" of others seem insignificant, trivial, or even silly. You can't believe people are upset, angry, or even concerned about such small matters.

One woman tells the class that when she complains about how some recent bad weather has kept her from going to meet a friend for lunch, her husband, a cancer patient, tells her in a very nasty tone, "I would give anything to have your problems!"

Patients and their caregivers in the room nod their heads as if to say, "Been there, done that." The woman seems surprised that others have shared similar experiences. Like many things we experience, we feel isolated and unique in our frustrations and even in our sorrows. Her husband, looking a bit guilty, then smiles when we all say we understand him. Completely.

Cancer patients and others who have experienced tragedy don't have much time or patience for other people's so-called problems.

Robert Fulghum, author of the book, *All I Really Need to Know I Learned in Kindergarten*, also wrote another short essay called, "Sigman Wolman's Reality Test" in which he defines the difference between a problem and an inconvenience. He uses a real-life experience he had as a young man when he worked at a resort in Northern California.

Fulghum describes how he made a mistake of complaining to a fellow employee about consistently bad food, wieners and sauerkraut, served several times a week. The man listening to him turned out to be a holocaust survivor.

Clearly, bad food, in fact any food at all, did not pose a significant problem to Sigmund Wollman who had survived Auschwitz.

After we discuss Fulghum's philosophy, I ask students to write about their problems and their inconveniences and how those might differ from the problems of people who do not have cancer or have not suffered great losses. Laughter fills the room again and again as each person cites an example. Dark humor results and would probably not be appreciated by the "untouched," those in our lives who consistently seem to worry about all the wrong things.

Healing Words

Problems or inconveniences? You decide.

Mother gets on my nerves.
Mother always talks about the past.
Mother doesn't remember who I am.

Doctor says I'm ill.
Doctor says I may need surgery.
Doctor says, "The cancer is back!"

My "ex" calls me all the time.
My new relationship isn't working out.
Karl left me when he found out I had cancer.

Having a bad hair day always depresses me.
I just can't believe my hairdresser cut my hair this short.
I'm having a no-hair day.

She had been terribly ill, but finally, she felt she had turned the corner. Elizabeth, 42, was being treated for advanced breast cancer. She telephoned her father to share some good news. What she heard on the other end of the line indicated more than a poor connection.

Phoning Home

I had just completed my third cycle of chemotherapy and was feeling strong and strangely buoyant despite the onslaught of drugs I was ingesting: Decadron, the steroid, the night before, Taxotere and the dreaded Adrigmycin chemo drugs the next day with more Decadron, Benadryl, and Zofran added to the cocktail. More Decadron and Zofran followed on the third day.

I had a slightly upset stomach and recurrent mouth sores but no nausea and no serious signs of fatigue. My hair was falling out by the handfuls, but even that couldn't dampen my spirits.

Feeling elated, I decided to call my father who lives in Europe to share my good news.

"Hey, how are you feeling?" was his first question.

"Well..."

I began to answer, but before I could continue, he interrupted with, "Good."

Then he proceeded to tell me all about his problems: the sprinkler system in the garden had broken, which meant that water had sprayed all night, soaking his plants.

Then his favorite English newspapers (he lives on an island off the coast of Denmark) had not been delivered to his home, causing him to make a special trip to the train station.

And, worst of all, his vacuum cleaner had broken.

"Can you imagine how difficult it is to get anyone to fix this kind of machinery on this remote island?" he asked me.

"Not really," I replied with detachment.

Thank goodness, I mused, I have problems in my life that can actually be solved rather than annoying little inconveniences that can take over your whole world.

— **Elizabeth Terry**

While confined to her hospital bed, Linda begins to envy those whose lives appear to be normal.

Problem-Free

At the hospital, during my darkest days, I remember gauging the staff's "happiness quotient" always comparing theirs to mine.

Truth was, I hated being so self-centered, hated having to discuss my every itch and pain and sensation, even though I knew my very survival depended on it.

In my delirium and fear, I was sure the staff had no problems.

"Look at them!" I'd think. "Laughing at their co-worker's joke, with their flowers and children's pictures on their desks. They are so lucky. And I am so NOT!"

— Linda Bergman

Bill's life and priorities changed with his transplant.

A Life-Marrow Transplant

Not too long ago, I thought the worst thing that had happened to me was discovering I had multiple blood-related diseases requiring a bone marrow transplant. A successful outcome could not be guaranteed, and a significant change of life would be required.

I had only a 60% expectation of survival, I would have to stay out of the sun for several years, and I would need medication for the rest of my life. As reality sank in, I realized that the best thing that had happened to me was discovering I had multiple blood-related diseases requiring a bone marrow transplant.

I've always been a marketer, optimistic about results, so I put my chances of survival at 100% and followed my wife's advice to "sell the business, liquidate all assets except our house, pay off all bills, retire, and spend time writing. Start by finishing the novel you've been working on for seven years."

Damn, what's not to like about that?

When faced with a life-threatening illness (I typically refuse to use the word cancer), some people change their priorities and some don't. Many are so caught up in their careers and lifestyles that, once diagnosed, they end up adding their illness and the requirements for recovery to their already long list of tension and anxiety producing "things to do."

This compounds the conflicts in their lives, intensifies the conflicts in their bodies, and, I believe, significantly lowers their chances for survival.

On the other hand, many (and I am one) put their illness first on the list and do everything possible to survive. This is an immediate and significant shift in priorities. What good is obtaining money, status, and possessions if you die before your never-ending quest is realized?

My priorities immediately changed to enjoying what I now had, actually somewhat less than before. In my case, less became more. I was able to focus on what remained and, to some extent, "see" it for the first time.

Prior to my illness, I had so many activities on my to-do list that I wasn't able to enjoy any of them, or even able to appreciate their accomplishment.

Now, with my illness under control, I take the time to enjoy whatever I'm doing, whether it is writing, gardening, getting together with friends, fishing, or traveling. I, like so many others, have been "reborn."

Hold a rose, smell it, and evaluate its construction for several minutes. There are countless more experiences awaiting me following what I now call my life-marrow transplant.

— Bill Matteson

In the midst of his treatment, Doug was putting every ounce of his energy into surviving his stem cell transplant so he could live, just live. He had learned what was important and what was not. He wrote the following poem about being in the hospital on an IV when he came to terms with his changed priorities and realized a recently ended relationship could never be rekindled.

Drops

While you were out getting your teeth whitened,
I dropped off my keys,
left them on your desk.
In the hospital there were no keys
no locks.
But there were the drips,
and I could
hear the drops
see the drops
smell the drops.
Like the rain falling now,
I can watch the rain
feel the rain
breathe the rain.
While you were out getting your teeth whitened,
I left your front door unlocked.

— Doug Wilkey

＜＜◆＞＞

When friends and family members telephoned Christine to see how she was coping while recovering from her first bone marrow transplant, she didn't always find their calls helpful.

Nobody's Home

One thing that cancer has taken from me is the patience to listen to gripes, groans, and gossip. The shock of diagnosis clears away the illusions of life. Suddenly, all that matters is family, friends, and love. To me, the only conversations worth having are those which are life affirming, not what was on television last night, how bad the traffic was on the way home, or how rude the person at the cash register was. Those are all trivial.

I used to allow people to dump on me. Now I realize that life is too short to listen to someone bitch about his or her co-workers.

Caller ID is a wonderful invention.

— Christine Pechera

It's Your Turn

In class, following the quiet time for writing, comments such as, "Gee, I don't know where that came from!" are not infrequent. Someone has suddenly written about a long-forgotten event or feeling. It has come from the depths of their memory. Then another person reads what he or she has written and again sighs, "I really feel better getting that out!" Psychologists have equated carrying around stressful or negative memories or feelings with loading ourselves up with a basketful of bricks. Each one is heavy. Once put in its proper place, or discarded entirely, we feel lighter, better. Whether you call it excess baggage or a load of bricks, you want to rid yourself of it as soon as possible.

Write about how your priorities have changed since you or your loved one experienced illness or tragedy. How did you feel before? What did you see as a problem then? What are your problems today? Are you able to relate in the same way to your friends or family members who are "untouched"?

Journalists use the idea of "compare and contrast" to show changes. The following sentences show you how to do that effectively.

Jump Start

Before ... I used to feel (angry, sad, frustrated) about ... and ... but now, I feel ... about ...

This changed when ...

Continue to describe the changes in priorities you have experienced and how those changes affect your relationships with others at work, at home or in social settings.

Chapter 9

Expelling Anger

Why do I have to die to rest in peace?
— Robert Prado

Each of us deals differently with anger. Some save it up bit by bit as the stress and frustrations mount. Then when it comes bursting out, often without warning, those around us may become targets of our harsh words, resentment, and even rage.

Add cancer or other tragedies to the equation and the results are often negative for everyone concerned. Some hold in their anger for decades, never acknowledging its presence or its building pressure. Family members and caregivers sometimes describe a sudden change of personality in those facing illnesses or other shocking news. People who first seem angry about their situations sometimes suddenly begin to over-control everything and everyone around them.

When patients or families describe the symptoms, I understand fully.

When you can't control your body (you have cancer) and you can't control how to cure your disease (doctors and caregivers prescribe and monitor your treatments) and you're too weak to do much (bedridden or on the couch), your mouth might be the only thing still working. And boy, do you work it!

"I suddenly became a world's expert on everything and everyone," Beverly told the class.

Bingo! That was me, too, and some might say it still is. I developed a bad habit — over-talking or interrupting others. I seemed impatient to get into conversations. After all, I got paid for talking as a teacher and found myself home and out of work while I was recovering from surgery. To make myself important, I had to butt in and get my points across.

I recognized that I was doing it, but I seemed unable to stop. I read an article stating that over-controlling conversations is a sign of insecurity usually based on anger issues. But I didn't feel angry per se. I also didn't want to be that obvious, feeling perhaps someone I knew had read the article, too, and might be analyzing me.

So I consciously tried not to be a know-it-all or an interrupter. I didn't completely solve the problem, but when I was with friends, I tried to at least take a breath once in a while to allow someone else to get their two cent's worth in during my silence. I could tell by the relieved looks on their faces that they were grateful.

When I described my problem in class, a male patient smiled and raised his hand. He began to speak. He told us about feeling especially angry about being restricted from driving due to weakness caused by his cancer medications; his wife was forced to chauffeur him from place to place.

"One day when she got out of the car and began pumping gasoline, I hollered lots of nasty advice out the window, telling her she was doing it all wrong. I felt she had taken away MY job, in other words, my personal role in life as simple as that might seem now."

I related to his comments, too. Not only did I tell my husband how to drive, I also told him how to fly. The fact that I didn't have a pilot's license and he used to be an Air Force instructor pilot in jets did not stop me from offering my opinion and my running commentary. Consciously now I try to keep my mouth shut. It works sometimes.

It may sound humorous, but it isn't even slightly funny for those spouses, friends, family members, and caregivers who find themselves walking a tightrope, trying to be supportive and helpful each day, while dealing with their own fears and frustrations. In addition to all that, they have to contend with an over-controlling blabbermouth.

Because of this syndrome, writing about anger seems to be a natural outlet for cancer patients and their caregivers. But, despite this, some of the class members still need a little coaxing. I notice this almost immediately when I give them the option of either writing about anger they might be holding in or the anger they have inappropriately let out.

This sneaky method is what's called a forced choice in psychology. You tell your child, "Do you want to clean your room first or mow the lawn first?"

No other choices are given.

Once I give students the forced choice of writing topics, adults routinely turn the tables on me.

"But, I'm not really a writer," one person protests.

"I've always hated to write. I don't even write letters!" says another.

"English was my worst subject in school," adds someone else.

Sometimes cancer patients can be a real pain. I smile, listen patiently, as patiently as I can, and then offer, "Well, maybe you never thought you had anything you wanted to say before. And, remember, what you're going through can really be told only by you. You're the expert on this. Only you know how you feel."

After we briefly discuss the topic of anger, I give the class 10 minutes to write about it.

I always wonder if anyone will be able to focus on such a personal topic and, if they can, given the short time, what the result will be. I also consider not asking anyone to share his or her writing, feeling it might be too personal. Writing about anger is one thing; sharing it by reading aloud is quite another.

To my surprise, when I tell the group to begin writing, pencils and pens begin working overtime. I think I can actually see smoke rising from some of their papers. Anger, it seems, is not really very hard to write about. Most participants do it eagerly and almost frantically.

Then, after the time expires, hands fly up all over the room. Everyone wants to read what he or she has written.

Healing Words

Here are some results from some so-called non-writers, the ones who, in some cases, have to be coaxed to write. Clearly, these are all individuals who have gotten in touch with their feelings and have let them escape onto paper.

In her job as an appointment scheduler for City of Hope, Annie, 50s, deals with cancer patients, scores of them each day. She is often the first person a new patient or family meets. She becomes very close to her patients and goes through the lows of their diagnosis and treatment and the highs of their successful outcomes. In her years there, she has gotten to know thousands of patients and their families. A divorced mother of two grown sons, Annie has lots of extra love to distribute along with the appointment slips. Although there are many schedulers, Annie's waiting line is always the longest as people wait for a hug, a piece of candy, or just a soft shoulder. Sometimes, though, her patients don't recover, and when someone like Sarah receives the worst possible news, Annie's arms

might be the first place they bring their anger, sorrow, or fear.
   Annie explains:

She Did Everything Right

She stood in my line, waiting patiently as she had done so many times before. She was returning from getting the results of her CAT scan. I could see by the look on her face that her visit with her doctor had not gone as we had hoped.

Sarah's usually bright blue eyes that always sought out others to help and encourage, were now red and swollen from crying, cast downward to the floor.

I finished scheduling the patient in front of her and, as he left, she rushed to my desk.

"Hey, girl, how'd it go?" I gently asked, almost stumbling over the question because I thought I knew what her answer would be.

I wasn't prepared for her response.

"Annie, I'm fucked!" she cried out as she shook her head. "It's in my liver and lungs and now I'm screwed!"

I stood and walked around to the other side of my desk to hold her as she cried.

"Why is this happening, Annie? I did everything right!"

As I thought of how to respond, I realized what her words meant.

She had indeed done everything right. She was a good, kind person who spent her lifetime always trying to help others. She took care of herself and was devoted to eating health foods. She was an athlete and a fitness guru. She was also doing exactly what her doctors and caregivers recommended. By those standards, she was leading a healthy life, doing everything in her power to get well.

But none of that mattered to the evil cancer that was now devouring her body. It is no respecter of persons. It preys upon whomever it wills.

Again she sobbed in her own defense, "I did everything right!"

"I know you did, Sweetie. I'm so sorry," I said softly.

I brushed her feathered blond hair behind her ear and cupped the side of her face in my hand. I encouraged her further by saying, "We'll get through this together."

It wasn't the first time I had made such a promise, and it won't be the last. As her body shook in my arms from her sobbing, I could feel the weight of the anger and despair in her tiny little frame.

I looked around the room at the other patients waiting to see their doctors and my eyes were met with compassion and understanding.

Even the patient who was next in line to schedule an appointment let me know with the tenderness in his eyes and his sad, knowing smile that he did not resent the delay.

— Annie Watson

I met Shannon, 33, in Colorado when I went back home for a family reunion. I told her about my Writing for Wellness class and we began emailing back and forth. She is married, works full time, and has two children in elementary school. She began writing to help her heal from being abused as a child. She chose poetry to help her vent her anger and frustrations about her childhood. She e-mailed me this poem.

The Smell of Lilacs

Morning arises with the smell of lilacs.
I awaken and I am free. Until night
When darkness comes with the smells
Of old sweat and clothes worn for weeks.
My bed is wet with terror.
My friend of freedom,

My sister of laughter, gone.
And the blackness sucks me in again,
These creatures who feed
From the purity within me.
I cannot move.
Then the waves make my stomach turn
And I am filled with terror,
Poisoned with stink and smothered
With the breath that tries to suffocate me.
I see a little girl.
Her friend of freedom, sister of laughter,
Are gone. No dreams to keep.
Only nightmares, until the lilacs come again.

— **Shannon Lynn Marshall**

When her class received the assignment to write about the anger they were dealing with, Edna spent exactly seven minutes (She timed it.) writing her poem. She did not explain what prompted her anger, and it wasn't until several classes later that she started, through more of her writing, to reveal its cause.

Why, Daddy? Why?

Why, Daddy? Why?
Why was I born?
Did you want me,
or were you forlorn?
Was I a bad girl?
Was I a burden?
Did I cry too much,

Or were you just hurting?
Wasn't I smart enough,
Or was I too smart?
I must not have been pretty.
Did I tear at your heart?
Did you want to love me,
Or decide not to try?
There's a pain inside me that cries,
Why, Daddy? Why?

— Edna Teller

After the group finishes writing about anger, Gordon, 70s, is one of the first to raise his hand. He begins by saying that he had been the sole caregiver for his life-partner, George.

Never to Hear His Voice Again

For someone who has never smoked and who was raised in a family of non-smokers, I view the so-called smoker's disease as a tragic waste of life.

Doctors said George, my partner of 28 years, officially died from congestive heart failure, but I know better. Smoking killed him.

Three times a day for four months I went to the hospital's Intensive Care Unit. It was the first place I stopped each morning on my way to my teaching job, the first place I went each afternoon on my way home, and the last place I visited just before going to bed. The nurses could have set their watches by my visits.

It was difficult.

I was angry. I was very, very angry. George shouldn't have been lying motionless, eyes closed, his throat pierced by a tube preventing him from ever speaking my name again.

I sat by his bed and read letters and cards to him. Over and over again, I read just so he could hear my voice even when he was sedated and sleeping — talking to him, touching his hand, his face, just letting him know I was there for him right up until the end.

I couldn't allow myself to cry at first, not until afterward, not until he was dead and I found myself alone for the first time in nearly three decades. I felt anger and a deep sense of loss.

I felt the anger and loss whenever I heard something on the car radio that I knew George would have enjoyed, too. I felt deep loss each time I heard a beautiful story about someone's gallant or brave deed, knowing George would have said, "Wasn't that wonderful?"

My best friend will not be forgotten nor will I forget his soft voice, a voice I never heard again — after they inserted the breathing tube.

— Gordon Dyer

Robin, 40, has an incurable disease, myelodysplasia with refractory anemia. At one point, she was on a path to receive a bone marrow transplant. She needed family members to be tested in a search for a possible match. If one were found, she might be able to return to a normal life. Unmarried and unemployed, she was desperate. Following the discussion about anger in their lives, her classmates began to write almost immediately. Robin stared at her blank paper.

Then, just as I told the group, "Take a few minutes more and then put down your pens and pencils," Robin started to scribble furiously. After just a few sentences, she put down her pen, sighed heavily, and raised her hand to read aloud. She read slowly and deliberately.

The class heard bitterness in her voice and saw tears in her eyes. When she finished, she looked relieved. Something significant had happened as she wrote those four sentences:

Dear Dad

You don't even care enough about me to pick up the phone to see how I'm doing or to find out if your bone marrow is a match for me! I'm mad, yes, but most of all I'm hurt each and every day. All I ever wanted in life was a dad who was going to be there for me.

And, oh, by the way, thanks for the defective genes, Robin.

— Robin Clarke

Christine was not a reluctant writer. She is a graduate of the USC Film School and had won awards for her writing. She has been writing since she was 10. Then, when her life seemed to be only positive, in her late 20s, in just a matter of months, she lost her health, her marriage, her job, and her life savings. Her younger brother, Rex, had already been lost to cancer at age 16. Her sister had also fought cancer. The following excerpt is from the journal Christine was writing during her original bone marrow transplant preparation and recovery.

February 13

I am so angry. My parents have sacrificed so much and worked so hard. They have already lost their eldest son to cancer. All their lives they have slaved for the good of their children, and now I am failing them, too. This is why I must beat this. I love Mom and Dad so much and I don't want them to ever become disappointed or discouraged. They deserve more than this from me.

My blood pressure is 88/44. I am sleeping most of the day. I am very tired and faint. Dad says my bone marrow is starting to die.

I am starting to die.

— Christine Pechera

Unlike others who find it difficult to put their thoughts on paper, Linda, a successful and well-known producer and screenwriter with numerous movies to her credit, makes her living writing for Hollywood. In the midst of producing her movie about Michael Landon's tragic death from cancer, Michael Landon: The Father I Knew, *Linda became exhausted from the 18-hour days of filming. She blacked out twice, found herself in an oncologist's office, and, on her 50th birthday, was diagnosed with chronic myeloid leukemia, an often deadly and highly aggressive form of cancer. Suddenly, she and Michael Landon had more in common than a movie. Linda also had a successful and supportive husband and two teenage children. Her body and mind were wracked with the effects of chemotherapy. Fear and anger consumed her as emotions welled up from the depths of her soul. Still, it seemed to her, that for most people around her, life was normal. Clearly, the world had not stopped just because Linda had cancer.*

The Anger

The worst part of being diagnosed with cancer is that dull ache of fear that totally permeates the mind and body. From the moment I woke, through the last minute of consciousness, day after day, terror reigned supreme. Now that's not news to any other survivors. We know now that fear is a given with a life-threatening disease.

With the fear comes resentment and anger and, for me, an uncomfortable self-centeredness.

I remember vividly wandering through the world wondering how everyone else could still laugh or play or dance.

I was dying from chronic myeloid leukemia for God's sake!

How could anyone still be happy?

— Linda Bergman

Following the writing and reading aloud, students often say they feel relieved and even somewhat tired. Expelling anger isn't easy or relaxing. Because it seems sometimes to come out almost explosively for some, several people have described letting out their feelings as being similar to setting off bombs they have been sitting on for much of their lives. As you write about anger, expect the unexpected.

It's Your Turn

If you are the cancer patient, the caregiver, the spouse, the friend, or a medical staff member, you have a unique perspective on anger and what is does to you and those directly affected. Also, some anger may not be related to having cancer at all, yet without expelling it, true healing may never take place. Likewise, if a catastrophic event has occurred, only you, the victim, family member, or friend have experienced the event in a particular way. Let out the anger by writing down your feelings and the details of what caused it. For healing to begin, you must get rid of the anger and resentment in your life. Writing about it is one place to start. Write the first words that come to mind. Don't hold back. If you want help getting started, use the words below.

Jump Start

I feel angry when I think about ...

Or, if you are angry with an individual, you may want to begin with:

You never seemed to ...

Even when I ... you ...

I get furious when I think about ...

    You may choose not to mail or deliver this message. Carefully consider the consequences of confronting another person with your anger. Be sure the time is right and, most of all, be certain that it is the right thing to do. Expelling your anger privately or reading what you've written to a close friend you can trust may provide enough relief.

Chapter 10

Forgiveness as Healing

My Lord teaches me
To forgive and forget.
Though the One who knows my heart
Knows I'm not able to do that yet.

— Annie Watson

Forgiveness is essential to wellness. We all have someone who needs our forgiveness. It might be a family member, a colleague at work, or anyone in our early or present life who we feel has deliberately hurt us. The greater the offense, the harder it is to forgive.

Asking for forgiveness from others makes us feel humble because in doing so, we are taking responsibility for our actions. We are admitting and "owning" the pain and heartache we caused others.

By forgiving someone else, we let go of the past and make a conscious commitment to free ourselves from the negatives in order to begin to heal.

Forgiving ourselves may be the hardest of all. When we carry guilt for some past action or omission, it can interfere with our healing. If we could live life over, we would undoubtedly do a lot of things differently.

Cancer patients and those who have suffered great losses in their lives tend to set new priorities. For many, having been faced with our own mortality, there seems to be an urgency to get on with life and to not sweat the small stuff. That may be the reason why the pencils and pens are not silent for more than a few seconds when students in class are asked to write about someone they'd like to forgive.

There is an old saying, "You cannot regret the words you do not say."

Granted, that adage is referring to words we might utter in anger or frustration, namely what we don't say will never have to be taken back or explained.

If words can help us heal, then we need to say them or write them. Of course, silently forgiving someone can be helpful sometimes. We often count to ten when we are about to blow our tops, but that may be merely a temporary delay.

However, there are words, words of forgiveness that sometimes need to be expressed directly to the individual we are forgiving. They may be read aloud or mailed to the person, or simply written for our eyes only.

The hurt we still feel could be related to something someone said or did to us as far back as elementary school or as recently as yesterday. It might even seem insignificant to someone else, but if we still remember it, chances are we need to take time to forgive. The pain may remain with us if we don't write about it.

A teacher's harsh words, along with the cutting remarks of childhood friends, may dominate our memories for years.

In my Writing for Wellness classes, students more often write about much more traumatic events than schoolyard nastiness.

Parents ask for forgiveness from a child, after they have knowingly favored his or her sibling.

Children ask for forgiveness for mistreating or disappointing a parent. When students write about forgiving someone, it most often involves one or both of their parents. Parents have the most influence over us, both positive and negative. Families are often in conflict, and the term "dysfunctional" did not come from thin air. We all know that some parents can damage children.

Also, sadly, child molestation is not an uncommon subject for forgiveness, because victims need to release their hurt, anger, and despair in order to heal. Something as serious as child abuse or neglect may not be easy to forgive or forget. Writing to the person and expressing the anger, disappointment, and loss of trust may help, especially when, in the end, you truly forgive them while still remaining true to yourself. This act of forgiveness on your part may actually empower you and help you begin to heal from the experience.

People you need to forgive may not even be alive. Or, perhaps, you may not know their present location. Still, it is important to write to them or about them.

Healing Words

When people forgive themselves, it usually is for something they did. In Joan's case, though, she needed to forgive herself for something she didn't do. As she read the following piece aloud in class, Joan choked up and had a hard time completing it. When she finished, she said she could no longer feel the weight of the psychological "baggage" she had been carrying around for more than 30 years. She told those who heard her read her explanation that she suddenly felt much lighter.

The $25 Regret

It has been more than 30 years since my father's death, and I didn't realize until just now that I have never really forgiven myself for something that was not my fault, and certainly not my wish.

Life in California was not good for us. Money was scarce and time was, too. Both my family and my husband's family still lived in New York. We saw them seldom, and I desperately missed having family close to me. In January, my husband's mother died, and we left our four children with friends while I accompanied him to her funeral. Also in January, my father retired and my parents moved to Florida.

At that time, there was a "triangle" airfare, which would have allowed me for just $25 to stop in Florida on my way back to California. I thought about it, but I was concerned about leaving our children longer than necessary. I had just seen my father in July, and while the money is not much by today's standards, it meant a lot to us then. I didn't go. My father died in February. As I traveled to his funeral, I recalled my father earlier saying, "You can always find money for a funeral. Instead, come for the good times."

I have tried to follow that rule ever since. Logically, I knew that my father never doubted my love for him, but emotionally I always felt I had done the wrong thing by not making that side trip to Florida.

Today I can see that in the more than 30 years of honoring his memory and his wishes, I have earned my forgiveness.

— **Joan Smith**

Before Robert read the following lines in class, he told us he had never fully forgiven his mother for holding him responsible, as the oldest son, for the bad behavior of his siblings while they were under his supervision. If something went wrong in their house, Robert always paid the price.

Mom

One thought came to my memory about growing up: the whippings by my Mom. Being the oldest of five, I was always the one to get punished. Apart from that, she was the sweetest person you ever knew or met.

Years later, after Mom died, I asked Dad about the whippings I got. He told me Mom was like that because at that time, during World War II, he had been called into the Army, had gone overseas, and was wounded in Germany. It was too much for Mom.

Now nothing can erase the memory of her being my Mom.

The only things erased now are the whippings.

— **Robert Prado**

In a previous chapter, Edna's poem about her father, "Why, Daddy? Why?" may have left the reader sad that decades later she was still suffering and holding on to her anger toward him. But, after her classmates wrote about forgiveness, Edna made a significant decision. Her explanation and brief letter shows her progress toward healing.

It's Time

I have chosen to forgive my father. What was his crime, you ask?

It was not one traumatic event. He didn't beat me. He was not an alcoholic or drug abuser. He owned a business, a kosher butcher's shop. His customers thought he walked on water. "How lucky you are," they would tell me, "to have such a wonderful father."

You weren't really there, were you, Daddy? You had no concept of who I was as a person. Your body was there, but your caring spirit was somewhere else, deep inside, hidden.

I forgive you, but not because what you did was right. I forgive you because, frankly, you've taken up too much of my energy, too much rent-free space in my brain. I forgive you, not for you, but for me.

By forgiving you, I free myself.

— Edna Teller

Joy was a victim of child abuse by family members and, for years, harbored resentment. Her poem shows a progression of her forgiveness and healing.

Help Me Forgive

Lord, drain the pain from out of my heart;
Let not bitterness be rooted there.
Pour down your love on smoldering grudge,
And still the breeze that fans the flames of hate.
Help me forgive as I have been forgiven.
Bring to Earth a little taste of Heaven.

— Joy E. Walker Steward

It's Your Turn

No one wants to be bitter; no one wants to hold on to past wrongdoings done to us or by us. A good start is to think about something that you need to write to someone who may have hurt you, knowingly or unknowingly. Just as we know cancer must be removed because of the damage it can to do our bodies, we know we must also rid our minds of the cancers of sadness, anger, and estrangement caused by holding on to negatives in our lives.

Write about who you would like to forgive. It could be yourself, a family member, a colleague at work, or anyone in your early or present life that you need to address. The person can be living or dead.

If you have trouble getting started, write them a letter.

Jump Start

Dear ...,
I forgive you for ...

Even though this is difficult for me, I have chosen to forgive you for ...

What you choose to do with what you write is not as important as writing it. Do this for your own health and happiness. To let anger and resentment lie within you is to allow negative feelings to determine your state of mind. Release those feelings and regain your freedom.

When you're finished writing your letter, you can hand deliver it, mail it, file it, or simply throw it away. One person in class burned his letter in his fireplace. As he did so, he said he saw his resentment vanish with the smoke. Decide what will be best for your own healing.

Chapter 11

Unfinished Business

You can snuff out my dreams,
but you can't stop my dreaming.
                        — Joy E. Walker Steward

Whatever pain has come your way, it hasn't arrived in a single day. Poetry aside, there is truth in that statement.

Students come to Writing for Wellness classes after having a variety of traumas. Some are recent, the death of a son in an accident, the loss of a spouse or parent after a short illness. Others are still dealing with how friends and family treated them very recently, perhaps during their diagnosis or recovery period. Some class members say that going through a divorce has caused a split in family loyalties and friendships as more than a marriage has ended.

Much of the pain they report experiencing, though, has happened over a period of time — family estrangement being one of the more frequent topics students write about.

Students also write about their own illnesses or those of their loved ones. And, thankfully, during the more than five years I have taught the class, most patients and their families experience triumph over diseases. Their writings reflect those passages in their lives. Others, however, record feelings of pent-up sorrow and anger as the disease starts to limit or ultimately end a life, sometimes theirs.

To think that merely writing about these tragedies once or twice would provide immediate relief is presumptuous. The suffering did not appear in a day nor will it be erased in one. After major surgery no one who is realistic expects a patient to leap from the hospital bed and run laps around the track. As everyone understands, it doesn't work that way.

Healing the soul and spirit may take even longer. For some, it may never happen.

Families are often torn apart over financial matters following the deaths of parents. Others, as we read earlier, were turned down by their own family members when they desperately needed their help. Conflicts over such life-and-death matters are not easily or quickly solved. That sense of betrayal may never disappear.

Sometimes students in class write their hearts out, literally. When asked to write about something that changed their lives, the pens and pencils start working and what often results concerns an unresolved issue with a family member, a friend, or a significant other.

In some cases, the writer has been a victim of a crime and may not even have known the perpetrator. Clearly, there is unfinished business that needs attention. Writing about these traumas may not immediately take away the pain, anger, or fear, but it may allow healing to begin.

Writing is a process just as healing is.

Healing Words

Rick's sadness and frustration erupted as he wrote about a serious family conflict.

Family Memories for Sale

My only brother threatened to serve me with a lawsuit to force the sale of a cottage that has been our family's summer retreat for more than 80 years.

I had been forewarned of the delivery of the legal documents, but until they actually came, I had held out some irrational hope that perhaps he might reconsider. He didn't. And that sobering missile delivered a prickly flush of betrayal from a figure I had held in esteem most of my life.

Big brothers carry the authority and power to emasculate younger ones. The fears of failure, of rejection, and of exposure were always in his favor when I was growing up.

"Are you chicken?" or "Get lost!" or "Mom, Rick swiped my..." or "I didn't bite holes in the toothpaste tube; it was the Squirt!"

With a brother six years older, I often felt that I had two fathers.

When I was in the sixth grade, he was off to college and practically out of my life. Yet, I still maintained a familial trust and admiration for a brother with whom I shared early adventures, memories, and relatives.

The carryover of striving to gain his approval stayed with me into adulthood.

Over the years, the responsibility for paying the family cottage's bills, handling of our mother's finances, and overseeing the care of our mother in the last six years of her life fell to me.

My brother's passivity was born more from my accommodation and his convenience than any rational division of responsibility. So my role as an enabler was established over time.

Now he wants his financial half of our summer home at today's bubble real estate values, forcing it on the market for liquidation.

This is incomprehensible to me. By announcing his intention to sell, my brother is dumping the fiscal and psychological future of the family house on me.

But each cry also has behind it the pleading of a family estranged by obligations of work, of school, of sports schedules so compelling as to preclude other gatherings during the year. The time for our family's repair, our renewal, our precious moments together comes only in our summer cottage.

What will enrich my brother leaves me poorer indeed, for it is the gathering of our families that is now up for sale.

— Rick Myers

(Since this writing, Rick has become the sole owner of the summer cottage, buying his brother's half.)

Annie told the group that for seven months she lived like a hostage in her own life. The fear, anger, and lack of control created by her situation was so intensely personal that she could not share its details with the class. She would only say it had put her entire life on hold. She felt robbed of her freedom and her peace of mind. Although she has not achieved complete forgiveness, she says that starting to write about the trauma and reading what she wrote about it in class has helped her begin the healing process. Her poem shows a lack of forgiveness and a private but continuing struggle to heal.

Unforgiven

What is it that's said about the evil men do
   and the good they leave behind?
For in the harm you brought me
   there's no good that I can find.
My soul belongs to God,
   my heart's mine to give away.

But the stain left on my mind
    for years and tears will stay.
The Poet has said the future's no place
    to place your better days.
But I run to those days to dim
    the memory of my bitter pains.
My Lord teaches me
    to forgive and forget,
Though the One who knows my heart,
    knows I'm not able to do that yet.

— Annie Watson

Ellen routinely drives her blind friend, Joy, to class. She seems painfully shy, but, if coaxed, she will accept a sandwich or bowl of soup after she gets Joy settled at a table with her Braille writer ready for use, her white cane secured beneath her chair, and her purse and papers appropriately stored. Then Ellen, carrying her own food, rushes out for her work at an elementary school children's program sponsored by the local YMCA. But one day Ellen stayed for class. The writing assignment dealt with unfinished business and the instruction was simple. Complete the sentence, "I still feel angry when..."

As soon as I presented the topic, Ellen began to write. She wrote and wrote without looking up once. What came out was a story that left us all feeling empathy and sadness for her and her family. Clearly there was still an open wound. She choked up and had to stop a few times as she read it aloud, but afterwards she said she felt much better as she started dealing with a loss she and her family had suffered years before.

My Niece Dena

I still feel angry when I think of my niece Dena. As I look back over our weeks spent here at City of Hope, I review the journey of a buoyant 26-year-old student nurse engaged to be married and fighting against a killer within.

Dena, at the time a nursing student at my alma mater, Pasadena City College, was attending a nursing class when she realized a lecture she was hearing on leukemia was painting a picture of herself. The symptoms being described were her own: fatigue, fever, malaise — symptoms that were consistently causing her to miss classes or leave class early.

Soon after going to her doctor, she was admitted to City of Hope. Day followed day. Test followed test. Family members stayed up night after night only to find that, at the end, Dena would not be a bone marrow-transplant candidate due to her own actions. During her years of "finding herself" she had experimented with and enjoyed smoking "pot" resulting in a chronic fungal lung infection that resisted all treatment.

— Ellen Lozar, RN

(Dena Lozar, the only child of Ellen's younger brother, died two months after hearing that lecture. Her fellow nursing students at Pasadena City College paid tribute to her at their graduation ceremonies.)

Over more than a decade, Robyn has had numerous serious and debilitating illnesses, the most recent causing her to have an operation, followed by plastic surgery. She could not work and found herself with no money and no health insurance. Then, a large tumor was found and thought possibly to be thyroid cancer.

She told the class that writing about her anger and fears has helped but has not begun to solve her problems. She said she would continue to write to heal, though. Her frustrations are evident in her writing as she searches for a cure and for peace of mind.

Relationships

Relationships. That's what matters to me most. Family, friends, church members, even strangers. I want them all to love me, just the same way I automatically love most of them — purely and from the soul.

Funny thing is, though, you can love people all you want, but it doesn't mean all that love will come back to you in the way you might expect.

The first thing you'll see when you run smack dab into a serious crisis is the sifting away of certain friends and even close family members. Chronic, serious, and mysterious illnesses can finally run off everyone around you, including your last best friend on the planet.

When the insurance benefits and "cash-ola" run out, you'd better have a disease others can brag about.

"Oh, my best friend has cancer!"

If you're not lucky enough to have that, you'd better have something that has the possibility of an early demise, or something that has at least been brought to light by Oprah. Nobody, and I do mean nobody, wants to hang around for very long unless your sickness can meet the requirements of being fully funded or, at the minimum, water-cooler-worthy gossip.

If you or someone you love gets in the crosshairs of an illness like one of the ones I've been through that have no clear-cut answers, you may find yourself sitting by a phone that doesn't ring or opening an empty mailbox. Unless you want to sink into a dangerous despair, you'd better know where to turn. In my case, I went straight to the top, the source of all power and light. God. Big miracles, little miracles are all around us. And what we need is a little bit of heaven right here on earth. Otherwise, the truth is, at the end of the day, you're all alone.

— Robyn Bryson

Robert, usually upbeat, could deal with his own pancreatic cancer, but he could not resolve his conflict about a sick baby.

Pain

I felt a pain.
The pain felt good.
I could live with that pain.
I did not want to live without pain.
Pain reminded me to slow down or stop.
All the pain I had after surgery,
Is erased from my memory now.
The only pain I still have,
Came when I was waiting for my turn at radiation,
And a nine-month-old cancer baby was ahead of me.
I still feel that pain and no pain killers
Will ever erase that.

— Robert Prado

It's Your Turn

Is there some event in your life that still makes you angry or sad? Do you have unfinished business with a relative, a co-worker, a neighbor? Have you been abandoned by friends during a crisis? What happened? Were you ill for a long time and then abandoned or was the abandonment part of a continuing process of estrangement from your family? As you write, be conscious of your feelings and include them. Remember, in writing to heal, the feelings as well as the facts must come out in order to be identified and dealt with. Use the sentences below if you find them useful.

Jump Start

After ... (illness, tragedy) ... my ... (friends/family/spouse) seemed to ... me and I felt ...

When ... (describe the incident) happened, I felt ...

I wanted to ...

Our family has never been the same since ...

Chapter 12

Bravest Hearts

I'm amazed how she's handling it. If it were me,
I'd be in the fetal position bawling my eyes out.
— Theda Clark

When Ruth came to my class, she was already weak, walking slowly and unsteadily. She came alone, carrying a brown-bag lunch, and immediately told the group she had driven herself from Santa Monica, more than a 40-mile round trip, right through the worst of the Los Angeles traffic, the center of town.

She had a slight grin on her face when she announced it, almost as if she were rather proud of her accomplishment.

She told us her age, 66, and her occupation, Hollywood writer, and mentioned in an offhand way that she had had "some successes" over the years. I learned later that she was responsible for several children's television shows. But her tone and attitude clearly indicated that she did not want us to pursue her comments about Hollywood. She seemed to have more important matters on her mind — her cancer.

I will never forget her words.

"I am here to learn how to express myself."

I immediately felt somewhat intimidated. This woman was an older and more successful writer. What could I possibly teach her?

Still, there she sat, pen in hand, ready for the day's lesson.

While students were finishing their lunches, I began to talk.

"Think about how having cancer has changed you, Think about the psychological changes as well as the physical ones. Then write about both the positive and negative aspects of those changes. Also, have you found new strength, new purpose?"

As a couple of hands went up and students offered some comments about how they had more appreciation for life and for their family members than before, Ruth sat stone-faced.

Although Ruth had people seated on both sides of her, she did not acknowledge them. Clearly, this was not a social event. She seemed totally focused on what she was about to do. When we ended the brief discussion and I asked students to begin writing, I saw Ruth hesitate for a few seconds and then begin to write at a furious pace hovering over her yellow legal pad. There was no doubt that she had a lot to say.

Soon she was joined by others in creating a special noise that teachers throughout the world know by heart — the symphony of pencils and pens on paper, a unique melody that emerges as the words flow and the desktops take on an extraordinary vibration.

A classroom of 50 creates a distinctly different sound from one of 25. An all-pencil group sounds different from an all-ballpoint one. Math students with their numbers sound different from the writing students who fire staccato-type notes as they end a sentence with a distinct dot, or when they cross their Ts with swift strokes. Those sounds truly are music to my ears. They mean people are spilling out words that are waiting inside them, waiting to explain, to thank, to forgive, or to free them of anger, sorrow, or frustration.

As I watched Ruth, I saw her write, sit back, write again, and finally utter a deep sigh. She obviously had finished her prelude, paused for the other players to continue the first movement, and then had taken up her instrument again to rejoin the symphony.

I hesitated to interrupt the music, but as their conductor, I felt I must.

"Take a few more minutes to finish that thought," I said. "You can continue to write after class or at home."

One by one, students stopped writing.

"Let's see what happened," I said.

I do not want students, especially those attending for the first time, to feel intimidated, so I don't ask anyone to read their work aloud. I continuously reassure them of that even before the writing lesson begins.

Once the pencils and pens are down, I ask if writing helped anyone. That gives a possible opening for the new or shy person who may want to participate to open up and talk about the process but not the product.

That day, Ruth's hand shot straight up.

"I'll read!" she announced rather than offered.

I was surprised. Not often does a newcomer volunteer so quickly. Most people ease into the process.

Ruth didn't seem to have time for that. As she began, her voice was soft, yet her words were beautifully and expertly assembled. This was obviously a woman who had a command of the English language far superior to anyone I had ever had as a "student."

"I'm dying!" were her first words. She said them as if she had just uttered them to herself for the first time. Several class members looked shocked as she continued.

I remember biting my lower lip, something I do almost automatically when I hear something very sad or dramatic in class and know I will have to speak when the reading stops.

"I'm dying!" she repeated.

Then, not in a sad or dramatic way but for the third time, she said,

"Yes, I am dying."

She did not cry, whimper, or even look distressed as she continued with, "but through this, I have come to understand what a wonderful life I've had."

She went on to summarize the highlights of her life — family, friends, career, and travel. I don't remember any specific words. I have forgotten those details. But I will never forget the expression on her face.

By acknowledging her life in its entirety, she seemed to gain strength and lose sadness. She seemed ready, ready to fight the cancer as long as she could, but also knowing the end had been predetermined.

When she finished reading, she sat back in her chair, eyes sparkling. No one spoke. A few people wiped tears from their eyes; others smiled at her in admiration. This was a strong woman and one who was facing her trials head on. Who would not be impressed with such resilience?

Ruth's bravery was admirable.

I stood, walked to her, and hugged her. She hugged back, but unlike other students on other days, no tears flowed from Ruth's eyes. She looked as if her mission had been accomplished and she was congratulating herself. Her body may have been weak but her spirit was intact.

Her writings are not in this book. She came to a few more classes and quietly wrote, never again sharing her words aloud. She always looked peaceful. Then, the last time she attended, she looked very weak, stayed only ten or fifteen minutes and as she stood and walked toward the door, she apologized, "I just had a treatment and I am too weak to stay. I'm afraid I will have to leave. Sorry."

Ruth died two weeks later.

If I could build a wall of heroes, Ruth's name would be on it beside the names of Christopher Reeve, Lance Armstrong, and Michael J. Fox whose battles with cancer and other medical challenges have been much more public. These are heroes known to the masses.

Ironically, though, in this era of "reality television," hundreds of thousands, millions even, wait with bated breath in front of their big-screen sets or handheld iPods to see an otherwise pretty dull person chow down on a bowl full of worms or swim in a slimy pool of snakes. Survivors?

Our country's viewers and indeed the entire entertainment industry are missing the boat. Instead of watching contestants motivated solely by greed who walk across a seemingly bottomless pit with only a safety rope separating them from death, why not meet the real heroes, the ones with no safety ropes?

Real-life survivors also eat worms, it's true, but almost always off camera.

These are people whose motivation is survival, all right, real survival. And, instead of lying and cheating their way through a fake contest, hoping that someone else fails, these admirable folks are surviving against all odds, fighting, and many times winning a real battle, such a the small boy I encountered for just five minutes.

My Hero, Rasheed

After my class Rick, Anna, Joy, and Carole were helping me clean up and pack up my car. I was rushed. We were chatting, laughing, hugging — the usual. As we went in and out of the main door, we passed by a very small boy, an African-American about seven I would guess, who was sitting in the lobby while his mother checked into the Hope Village where long-term patients and their families stay in cottages.

She looked young, perhaps in her mid-20s. It is routine to see people checking in, so I went about my business. Then my attention focused on the young boy who was wearing a surgical mask, a wool hat pulled over his bald head, a very heavy coat, long pants, and sports shoes. He looked like he was dressed for a Michigan snowstorm, not for a sunny 75-degree California day.

My first glimpse was of his skin, not a healthy color, but a gray tone, not like anyone I had seen before. Not much of his skin was even showing, only his small hands and a bit of his forehead. His big brown eyes stared up at me. He looked afraid, but much more, he looked cold, chilled. He was shaking, almost uncontrollably.

As soon as I saw him, I remembered we had been given Easter baskets handmade by a dear friend of mine, Beverly Melrose, from the Seattle area. She made each one with a handle and Easter bunnies done in needlepoint on the sides. She mailed them to me so I could give them to participants during class. I had put Easter candy in each one. Beverly had made 20 of them. We had three left.

When class was over, we encouraged one man to take two to his granddaughters and another man took one to his wife, a patient too ill to attend class. When I looked back in the room, there were none left.

Then I saw Anna's. It was there on the table with her purse. Without a word from me, Anna picked up her basket and took it out to the boy as he sat alone and sad. She smiled at him and said, "This is from the Easter Bunny!" as she handed it to him. His eyes lighted up and he pulled his mask down for a second to utter a weak, "Thank you."

I saw Anna, herself a colon-cancer patient, disappear back into the classroom, away from my sight. I later found her in there, tears streaming down her face. When I whispered to her that it was a lovely gesture, she whispered back, "I would have given him much more if it was in my power to make him well. I came back in here because I didn't want him to see me in tears."

Then, as I started getting ready to leave, I remembered I had a handmade "surgeon's hat" with wild colors that was made by another friend of mine, Carla, to cheer up leukemia children who are bald and undergoing chemo. She made them in different sizes and colors — but there was just one other exactly like the one I still had.

Around Halloween I had given all of the others, except one, to Jeanne Lawrence, thinking the hospitalized kids might enjoy "dressing up" like doctors.

I had given the matching one to my plastic surgeon, Dr. Andersen, who told me he loved it. They are expertly made and are reversible with contrasting colors inside.

A retired nurse, Lillian, who is in my YMCA swim class, had asked me for a pattern so she could also make some hats for City of Hope patients and I had given her one of Carla's. That April day, more than five months later, Lillian gave me back the hat, the twin to Dr. Andersen's and somehow I had mistakenly brought it inside with my other items for the class.

I picked up the hat and went back out into the lobby with it. I asked the boy his name. He pulled down his mask and weakly replied, "Rasheed," as he continued to look at the tiny basket and examine the candy and chocolate eggs inside. He didn't eat any of the sweets. In fact, he didn't look like he wanted to eat anything at all right then, but he held on tightly to the gift just the same.

Then Anna came back out to the lobby with a yellow plastic bracelet. Again, we had just one of those left in the classroom. She presented Rasheed with it and told him it was just like Lance Armstrong's.

I added, "Lance beat cancer and you will, too."

Rasheed nodded his head. He seemed to know about Lance Armstrong.

Then I showed him the colorful hat and asked him if he would like to have it, telling him there were only two like it — one was given to a doctor in the hospital.

"You'll have the only other one," I assured him.

Again his eyes lighted up, he nodded and reached for it. But, before I gave it to him, I went to his mother, still writing and writing, as she stood at the counter. It seemed odd to me that it was taking her so long to check in.

I asked her if it was okay to give him all those items.

She said nothing. She kept writing with her head down. Then the woman at the reception desk said to me, "She's deaf. She doesn't hear you. Her son will have to translate for you."

My heart sank. That tiny boy with cancer had more troubles than many of us would have in a lifetime. What was taking his mother so long was that she had been writing notes back and forth to the receptionist, asking her how the Hope Village operated so she could help her son get well. She, too, had more troubles than many of us will have in a lifetime.

I picked up a pen and paper and wrote my question to her, asking her if it was okay for Rasheed to have the things. She read the note and nodded and smiled, tapping her heart and signaling her thanks.

A few minutes later they walked out together, hand in hand.

Many unforgettable moments have happened in that classroom, in that building, on that campus.

Meeting Rasheed and his mother was the most recent one.

When I ask students to write about their hero, it doesn't take long for them to begin. Funny, but nobody ever writes about a rock star, a movie star, or Donald Trump.

Healing Words

Chakib "Chuck" Sambar, 60s, a friend, a college professor, elected school board member/president, and a former high school principal, substitutes for me when I have surgery or cannot teach Writing for Wellness classes. Cancer has touched his personal life in many ways.

Three Women

I want to describe my dinner with three beautiful and inspiring women. My first dinner companion was Vickie, 40, who was married with no children. She had a round face, sparkling and seductive brown eyes with long eyelashes, a very warm personality, and a smile that made one comfortable and at ease. She was sensitive, an attentive listener, and a very caring person. She had worked as a doctor's receptionist.

My second companion was Joanna, a professional young woman who worked as a chiropractor and nurse. She was single, slightly younger than Vickie, had a sparkling and vibrant personality, an effervescent smile, penetrating brown eyes, and a great sense of humor. She wore a chic black hat and black pants with a simple white blouse.

My third dinner companion was the love of my life for 38 years, my wife, Mary, a warm and loving grandmother of our only grandson, Nathan. Mary had prepared a gourmet dinner, set a colorful table with a lovely spring bouquet, chilled a bottle of Chardonnay wine, and baked a peach cobbler.

Before dinner, the women chatted. Joanna wanted a glass of water, while Vickie and Mary threw caution to the wind and asked for wine. The three conversed, laughed, and compared notes on their latest encounters — slow-growing hair, loss of breasts, and their latest reactions to medications.

All three were cancer survivors who were battling their second or third bouts. I listened as Joanna said, "My life with cancer is like traveling on a train in a dark tunnel. I started with one group of friends and, as I get closer to the end of the tunnel, I have a new group."

Mary added, "When I meet people who were my friends, they don't know what to say. They are really ill at ease to call or talk to someone who is fighting to stay alive."

"My friends feel very uncomfortable talking to me. Their way of dealing with my problem is to ignore me," Vickie said.

All agreed that their experiences with cancer had changed their lives, their friends, and the way they viewed their relationships. In their desire not to burden others, they chose to be with those who knew and understood. They derived more comfort, support, and empathy from those who had traveled their path, felt their pain, survived their struggle, and kept positive and hopeful mental attitudes.

They understood the meaning of a lost breast and the scarring of their bodies. They understood the meaning and significance of a CAT scan, stem cell transplant, infusion, chemotherapy, and collapsed veins. They also knew that survival required strength from those around them.

All three beautiful ladies agreed that the last thing they wanted was for someone to feel sorry for them. They wanted someone who would listen patiently with a sense of optimism. All of us can help by knowing that among those who wage the battle with cancer, their experience is intensely personal, painful, inspirational, and heroic. Yes, heroic. I thank my dinner companions for taking me into their circle of love and friendship. They shared their feelings, opened my eyes, and made me feel wonderful about being loved and accepted by them. There was much more to that dinner than good food and fine wine.

— Chakib Sambar

(Since Chakib wrote this, his wife, Mary, and her two friends, Joanna and Vickie, have all passed away.)

While her mother, Donna, continued to battle for her life after receiving a stem cell transplant, Lindsey, 12, wrote this poem, having already seen her mother fight cancer for two years. Clearly, Donna is Lindsey's hero.

She Fights

She fights today; she fights tomorrow.
She fights even as she goes through sorrow.
She fights strong; she fights tough.
Some even say that she fights rough.
She fights all week. She fights all month.
In my mind, she is really buff.
This fighter is indeed my mom.
She fights her cancer very strong.

— Lindsey Logan

Jeanne's heart had to be doubly large to endure what others could only imagine. Bill writes this tribute.

Heart to Heart

When I consider a bravest heart, I think of a lady whose daughter had leukemia. She was there as Michelle, 8, went through chemotherapy. She also administered medications, witnessed the resulting traumas of hair loss and puffiness, and suffered through her child's pain and hospitalizations.

Out of her deep love, she persevered for nine years until that battle was lost when Michelle was 17.

Recovery from the loss of her daughter came hard and is still in progress.

This woman is my bravest heart.

Is it only because of what she went through with her daughter? No, she is my bravest heart because she also went through it a second time. With me.

Jeanne and I had been married only six months when doctors told me I needed a bone marrow transplant due to pre-leukemia.

I knew it was a devastating blow to her, but I never heard her ask herself, "Why me?" Nor did I hear her complain, saying things like, "I've already paid my dues. I've been through enough. I can't face going to a hospital again; it's too painful!"

No, I never heard that.

What I heard was, "Okay, we're going to face and beat this together. Then you're going to concentrate solely on getting well."

She took over, arranging for all the duties of life, the bill paying, the housework, the yard, everything, in addition to taking care of me. Everything was on her shoulders. There were no complaints, no tears, no personal thoughts. She was with me 24/7, and she orchestrated my recovery like a maestro.

Who do I think of as a brave heart? My wife is a brave heart, and hers is the closest heart to mine.

She lost once, yet faced a second challenge head-on. So far, we've won, but then it hasn't been nine years yet either.

— Bill Matteson

(At this writing, Jeanne was taking care of her mother who had been diagnosed with cancer.)

Annie says her heroes are people she sees at City of Hope every day, those who wait in her line to check in for or make their doctors' appointments.

She first wrote and read this in Writing for Wellness class. Then she was asked to re-read it to an audience of 900 patients and family members gathered in an auditorium on Survivor's Day.

There were very few dry eyes.

My Daily Dose of Inspiration

People often ask me if it's hard to work at City of Hope. "Doesn't it get depressing having to see people so sick with cancer every day?"

Not everyone will understand my answer. I love my job. I can't imagine working anywhere else. What makes it so special for me are the very same patients who others wonder about. The City of Hope patients are my daily dose of inspiration.

For ten years, I have watched them walk through those doors, each with their own story to tell of loved ones at home, lives put on hold — some even making their long journey completely alone.

Every story is different, but with one thing in common. Their lives have been interrupted and redirected to this unknown place to fight a battle they didn't choose, a battle for their lives.

They come not knowing what to expect and they find a routine of seemingly endless waiting and uncertainty and, sometimes, pain. But they also find a team like nowhere else, that gives them hope when no one else could, their doctors.

They are our angels in lab coats.

The patients also find something they may not have ever dreamed they possessed. They find the strength, courage, and dignity of their own human spirit. And it is from their strength, courage, and dignity that I am inspired every day. They smile, make jokes, and sometimes share their hearts with me.

I hold each one of them in my heart and remember them in my prayers.

— Annie Watson

It's Your Turn

Who are your heroes, your role models? Think about why you value them and what they have done in their lives or their struggles to inspire you, to motivate you to fight on. Are your heroes nationally known figures? Are they your friends, neighbors, or fellow survivors? Write as specifically as you can, giving details about the who, what, when, and why of your admiration for them. To get started quickly, you may want to use the suggestions below.

Jump Start

The first word that may come to your mind is your hero's name. It will make an easy start.

... is so brave. I have felt this way from the day I saw/heard about him/her and how he/she ...

When things get bad, I always think of ... because ...

After you write, consider giving/sending your finished product to your hero. Can you imagine a better way to honor him or her?

Chapter 13

Heroes and Helpers

There is no profit in curing the body if, in the process, we destroy the soul.

— Samuel H. Golter, CEO
City of Hope 1926-1953

Often in my class, cancer patients are focused on their own small world of recovery. Their round-the-clock contacts are with medical personnel and their other interactions are with their family caregivers and friends, their team of supporters who have rallied around them.

When the patients get well enough to attend classes, they often are still in awe of those who helped them during those dark days. Poems, thank-you notes, essays, and letters come easily from them as they look back to times when they may have been too weak or too preoccupied with their own health needs to acknowledge those who helped pull them through.

Medical personnel, too, are often busy helping save the patients. There is little time to stop to put an individual patient's life into perspective. Later, they may share stories about how much they learned from witnessing triumph over tragedy.

One of my personal heroes is Dr. Lucille Leong, my oncologist. After all of the lab test results have been examined, the x-rays screened, and the treatments prescribed, she takes time to see each patient as a person, each family as individuals. She is smart, sensitive, and humorous. Besides, how many doctors always take time to give you a hug?

In addition to treating me for cancer, she became a personal medical mentor who worried about my raging psoriasis, which showed up after the cancer. She saw the frustration a chronic skin problem was causing and recommended a dermatologist, Dr. Janice DaVolio, who has worked miracles to solve the psoriasis problems. Dr. Leong does this for all of her patients, which is why she is exhausted and wrung out from caring for everyone but herself.

I ask doctors, nurses, and staff members at City of Hope who attend my classes to write about their experiences working at a cancer center, interacting daily with the ill and, sometimes, the dying. I ask who they admire and why. Their heroes are most often their patients.

I also ask the patients in class to write about their heroes. Their heroes are the medical staff — the doctors, the nurses and those unseen researchers in their laboratories searching for cures.

Here are some stories from the many sides of the cancer experience:

Healing Words

Students in class are given an assignment to experiment with word repetition as a writing technique. I use Martin Luther King's "I Have a Dream" speech as an example of effectively repeating the same word or phrase to begin each sentence. The topic for the writing is their choice. Using that technique, Carole, bald and still wearing a surgical mask to class following her double stem cell transplant, chose to pay tribute to her nurses. She later printed out her words on stationery with a colorful ice-cream-cone background and the poem was published in City of Hope's newsletter Hope Notes. *Nurses have passed the poem on to colleagues in several Los Angeles area hospitals where it remains posted in the nurses' stations.*

Here are Carole's words.

We Are Here for You

I've always known that nurses were a competent, courageous, compassionate crew. But until recently, I never discovered just how truly amazing each one was. Like yummy ice cream, nurses come in an assortment of wonderful flavors.

Some nurses exude confidence as they coordinate and juggle dozens of tasks with the greatest of ease.

Some nurses inspire with a glowing smile and a warm hello.

Some nurses breathe life into your weary soul with such affirmations as, "You can do it! You're doing good! You're where you should be."

Some nurses say it's going to be okay and, somehow, when they say it, you know that it will be, too.

Some nurses are like mother hens and are constantly reminding you to press on as they say, "Remain calm. Get some rest."

Some nurses administer healing power by softly singing rich songs of gospel praise.

Some nurses applaud you when there has been a positive change in a lab report.

Some nurses listen, really listen, when they ask, "How are you?"

Some nurses show empathy with a tear or two.

Some nurses give you a gentle, reassuring touch — over and over again.

And, sometimes, a nurse is a traveling nurse who spontaneously appears at a moment of crisis, bringing stability and relief, then suddenly vanishes — leaving one wondering, "Was I just visited by an angel?"

— Carole Palmquist

Without Shirley's blessing on Writing for Wellness class, it might not have become a reality. Unlike others who work in institutions heavy with administrative bureaucracy and paperwork that sometimes prevent rather than assist, Shirley cut to the chase. In just a few days, she had reviewed the course objectives and teaching methods and given the signal to begin classes. She attended the first session and many others over the years. She has been a clinical social worker, program developer, and research specialist at the City of Hope for 15 years. She developed a pilot project (Transitions Program) to offer enhanced support services to those facing end of life and bereavement. Psycho-educational interventions included individualized patient and family counseling and support groups, personally touching hundreds of lives. Often in one-on-one sessions, Shirley and the seriously ill patient come together to evaluate options. Shirley has touched hundreds of lives. These encounters are the inspiration for this poem.

Soul Work

Your strength humbles me.
I stand at the door and take a deep breath,
A prayer for wisdom, courage, compassion, guidance,
Unsure what the next hour will bring.
You smile as I enter,
Ever optimistic that those who work here offer hope.
You tell me what matters, who is involved,

How your days are interrupted by this disease,
The dread you feel with each scan, test, blood draw.
You tell me of your loves, your unfinished dreams.
I tell you of next steps and decisions to be made,
Consequences and choices, implications.
We explore uncharted terrain.
Exhausted, we part.
Your strength humbles me.

— Shirley Otis-Green, LCSW

Like Shirley, Jeanne is also on the front lines. Each day it is her job to meet patients at the Patient/Family Resource Desk and introduce them and their families to all of the programs and facilities City of Hope has to offer. She helps set up support groups, gets the word out to potential participants, and then networks with families and medical personnel. Each day she also provides hugs, smiles, and prayers for all involved. As one person leaves her arms, another approaches. Over the 34 years she has worked at City of Hope, she has met and become close to thousands of patients and their family members. A cancer survivor herself, Jeanne's own life has not been untouched by tragedy and illness. The oldest of her three sons, Tim, was injured in an accident and became a paraplegic at the age of 30. He recently died. Her words describe what Jeanne learned from one special patient.

We Learned from Each Other

My story began in the early part of 1973 when I decided after being home six years raising three young boys that I was going to rejoin the work force. My husband, Bob, thought I should stay home a while longer, but I convinced him that things would be all right and to just give me six months to prove myself.

Now, 34 years later, I think I successfully convinced him it was the right thing to do. From my first day at the remarkable City of Hope Cancer Center, my heart and life have never been the same, primarily because of the philosophy outlined close to 90 years ago by one of its founders, Samuel Golter. "There is no profit in curing the body if, in the process, we destroy the soul."

The tenacity of our patients to conquer and survive catastrophic illness also provides a continuing lesson that has particularly touched me. I have had the privilege to know patients and caregivers alike during my tenure. Recently it occurred to me that every single patient has a specific need and also a special story to tell. Some stories are happy, some sad, but more often than not, there is a remarkable strength and courage that emanates from each person and their unique story.

A wonderful gentleman about 40 shared his unforgettable story with me. He began by telling me that he was thankful that his cancer had recurred after his second bone marrow transplant. He immediately noticed that I was a bit taken aback by this comment. He quickly explained that before his cancer battle, he had been quite successful in business, earning a great deal of money.

Then cancer struck and everything in his life began to change. He could no longer work and had to undergo the transplant. After a very short time following his transplant, his cancer returned. That meant he needed a second one. Unfortunately, that transplant also failed and he was in relapse. There were no further treatment options open to him and he knew there was not much time left. But he was positive about his journey.

He told me, "Before I came down with cancer, my primary goals in life were to keep working to make more and more money for my family."

"But now I'm aware of what is really important in life — my relationship with God, spending time and enjoying my wife, children, and friends. I can see clearly what beauty the trees, flowers, mountains, and oceans offer."

"I took so many things for granted. I thank God every day for these blessings."

I will never forget his words or the lesson they carried. I, too, want to remember to thank God every day, especially for patients who share their stories and give me insight into what life is really about.

— Jeanne Lawrence

Marilyn, a registered nurse who worked 12 years in pediatric oncology, is currently an oncology resource nurse. She attended Writing for Wellness classes for more than a year and still comes when her schedule permits. She writes here about one tiny patient who she and her colleagues will never forget.

Miracle Child

Octavio, the eighth son, the baby, in a large Mexican family, was diagnosed with leukemia when he was only eight months old. Somehow his parents found their way to City of Hope, and we all did our best to help this little boy survive.

Childhood leukemia is quite curable today, but babies are considered at very high risk and often suffer grave side effects from the intensive therapy.

Despite our love and care, Octavio developed a serious blood infection, seizures, and even had a stroke when he was just two years old. He had difficulty seeing and hearing, could not walk or talk, and spent most of his time sleeping or being pushed in a stroller by his attentive mother.

Octavio's family lived on a ranch in Mexico and worked with horses.

Once the staff learned this, everyone brought him toy horses, and he had a little cowboy hat and cowboy boots.

But no matter how hard we all tried, he failed to show any emotional response, even though his physical condition had improved and his leukemia was in remission.

One of the nurses, who owned and rode horses, decided to try "horse therapy."

She brought one of her horses by trailer to the hospital and led it into the pediatric play yard behind the young boy's hospital room. Octavio's mother and father brought him outside in his cowboy gear and lifted him onto the horse.

His father held him on while the nurse walked her horse around in a circle. Before long, a smile appeared on Octavio's face, and he actually laughed out loud.

This was the turning point in Octavio's remarkable recovery. He started speaking and learned to walk again. He completed his treatment and eventually went home to Mexico to live on the family ranch.

We lost track of him for a few years but, one day, his entire family appeared in the clinic with then eight-year-old Octavio — the picture of health, a shy smile on his face, and dressed from head to toe as a small cowboy!

Being a pediatric oncology nurse has its joys and rewards, and even though some outcomes are not good, most are. The pluses far outweigh the negatives.

Children are resilient, optimistic, accepting, joyful, trusting, and they have the remarkable ability to be in the moment. They do not dwell on the past or anticipate the future, and those of us who care for them during catastrophic illness have learned to be like them. They feel pain and they cry, of course, but they smile easily, hug generously, and forgive readily.

We make it through the difficult days and years because we

remember Octavio and all of the miracle children who have touched our lives forever.

— Marilyn Rhodes, RN, BSN, OCN

It's Your Turn

Who has been a hero or helper for you? A friend? A spouse? A doctor or nurse?

Think about how you have felt in the depths of your sorrows or fears. Write about who hugged you, listened without judgment, and reassured you that they would be there for you. Include as many of your feelings from that time as you can remember. Use the sentences below to help you get started.

Jump Start

... is my hero because ...

Dear ...,
It has been (months, years) since ... but I will never forget how you helped me when ...

Write about what the person's loyalty and strength meant to you. Describe what happened and how the person helped pull you through. Send them what you write.

Part III

Getting on With Your Life

Chapter 14

Gifts and Blessings

God blessed me just the other day,
Gave me a second chance, showed me the way.
— Janet Gray

Janet looks at her second bout of cancer, non-Hodgkin's lymphoma, and her stem cell transplant as her second chance at life. It has been nine years and she still considers it a gift.

What one person might view as a blessing, someone else might see as a curse. What they both might agree on, though, are the words, "It is better to give than to receive." The irony is, of course, you receive far more in return by giving.

Gifts can be physical, material, or spiritual. In some phases of life you may value some over others. Sometimes your physical gifts of health and mobility are taken for granted until you lose them. When you think back to a time in your childhood when you broke a bone and had to be in a cast for a few weeks, you remember how you missed your mobility. You remember the previous days or weeks when you took it for granted that you could walk, run, throw.

During cancer treatment that realization is magnified a hundred-fold for some. In the depths of cancer treatment and recovery, material goods take a back seat to the "gift" of receiving a good lab report or hearing that your chemotherapy has been completed.

Spiritual gifts of prayers by friends or family provide comfort and peace of mind. Your own religious faith may be a gift of reassurance and direction in your struggle to survive. While some gifts are profound, others are simple. My gifts to students in my classes are in the latter category.

One part of my life that has given me joy and one that millions of other men and women can relate to involves the preparing and serving of food. I have always received great satisfaction from the entire process, whether it was cooking for family and friends or taking home-baked treats to neighbors or to work for my colleagues and students.

Having the opportunity to combine two activities I love — teaching and feeding people — sometimes seems too good to be true, and now Writing for Wellness has become Eating for Wellness, too. What began as a gift to my writing students has become a blessing in return.

I was asked to move my writing classes to the daytime in order to accommodate more people who were on campus during business hours. We settled on noon as a starting time, believing that patients usually weren't scheduled to see doctors between noon and 1:00 p.m. and staff members also would be free to attend during their lunch hours.

But immediately I wondered, "What will I feed them?"

The question was never, "Should I feed them?" because I had already clearly established my philosophy of "breaking the ice by the breaking of bread."

I witness in my classes that students relax and bond when they eat. It is a fact. Food soothes and disarms. I have also been told I was probably a Jewish mother in a previous life. Clearly, I am not happy when people aren't eating — and eating.

When Fullerton College had student celebrations on the grassy quadrangle outside my classroom, I would don my rubber gloves and paper hat to join other faculty members dishing out everything from ice cream to tacos as hoards of hungry kids lined up on that 22,000-student campus. I learned from those experiences that the gift of free food and a smile always results in a returned smile and a grateful thank you. What could be better?

Therefore, the idea of "catering" a meal for a dozen or more writing students each week excites me. My lesson plans for writing assignments are tried and true. What works in the evenings works at noon. But, once told about the time change for class meetings, I realized I had to get busy planning my menus. Chicken soup seemed to be a natural at first and it has quickly become a tradition. Unless it's 90+ degrees in the California shade, it's the staple. Call it soul food, call it comfort food, or just call it part of our culture, few people ever turn it down. Various salads, sandwiches, fruit, and desserts fill out the menu and fill up the participants.

At first, students often comment, "Oh, you shouldn't have!" but I can see by their enthusiasm that they are grateful. Later they tease me with comments, "What? No chocolate-chip cookies? You're slipping!" or "No fresh pineapple? No tip!"

Some patients preparing to undergo a bone marrow or stem cell transplant often arrive wearing surgical masks and armed with instructions to avoid certain foods. They also sit apart from others to prevent any possible contamination. Everyone understands.

But other patients who are encouraged to increase their intake of calories and find themselves without an appetite at home report looking forward to our class lunches.

"I couldn't eat a thing at home," Carole Palmquist said wearing her surgical mask and looking thin and pale at the first class after her transplant. After a few minutes, though, she had a half-filled bowl of soup and a few small items on her plate. Before long, she had returned for seconds and joined the group as they all chatted and ate.

I get such satisfaction watching them enjoy their meals as they make conversation and then write about their lives that the schlepping of pitchers, platters, and plates to and from my car seems insignificant.

Food is indeed a gift. Being able to enjoy a meal is something cancer patients look forward to and recognize as a sign of their recovery.

Another "gift" cancer patients receive is that of cancer itself. It sounds grim and impossible to the untouched, but many cancer patients and survivors nod their heads when the subject comes up. They understand completely.

I addressed 800 cancer survivors as a guest speaker on Survivor's Day at City of Hope with these thoughts:

The Secret Gift of Cancer

Following my first bout with cancer, I wrote a short story in which a woman told by doctors that she is dying, suddenly and dramatically begins to look at the world — her family, her friends, nature, and even everyday problems — in a new light. The tragic news she receives causes her to reevaluate everything she does. Everything.

Having cancer can be like that. Suddenly, the blue of the sky seems bluer when you think you may not always see it. Even a rainstorm or a cold, windy day may seem beautiful in new ways. Your family and friends become more precious than ever before.

What you might have previously viewed as a problem is seen as merely an inconvenience. A car that breaks down, a bad hair day, stress at work, or arguments with family members all take their rightful places as minor annoyances. You wonder why you ever wasted precious moments on such trivialities.

Life and death. That's what matters. Love, faith, friendship, music, learning, and understanding. Cancer suddenly separates the important from the meaningless.

Toward the end of my short story, the main character learns these valuable lessons as she sees her numbered days begin to slip away. She lives every second, every minute to the fullest, thankful just to be alive. Then, when she is preparing to die, her doctor realizes a mistake has been made and apologizes to her, saying her tests were mixed up with another patient's who has almost her exact name. The main character is actually perfectly well. She was never ill. She has been given another chance at life.

I often tell people that surviving cancer is like receiving a gift. It is a gift you didn't ask for and one you can't return. It is one you would never want to pass on to anyone else, but one that can transform you forever in deep and positive ways, allowing you to live each hour, each day you have, with a new and more meaningful perspective. A gift, indeed.

Healing Words

Students in class receive copies of my speech "The Secret Gift of Cancer" and then write about how they view the special gift many of us share. When I ask what they value most, people who have survived cancer or other tragedies rarely mention material gifts. Most often they write about their new life-changing perspective.

My dear friend Lois and I taught high school together for years before she went on to become a principal and I got a position as a college writing professor. Our husbands, both engineers, became friends, too, and our families routinely shared holiday celebrations since our parents all lived out of state. Lois and her husband Bill both got cancer at the same time. Lois has taught my class for me from time to time over the five years and brings a special perspective, having been both a patient and a caregiver for her spouse.

Blessings and a Gift

My advice to anyone who has or has had cancer is to remain alert for a blessing or unexpected gift that might come your way. I am a 15-year survivor of ovarian cancer, which included three surgeries and four rounds of chemotherapy. And, during that time, I also lost my husband of 39 years to cancer.

However, I am so thankful that I seemed to have been given unexpected blessings, a positive attitude, loving family and friends, and an ability to keep going "no matter what." But, one gift I received I never dreamed as a possibility or a reality.

Before I describe my unexpected gift, I want to tell you a story. A very dear friend of mine, Mary, passed away from cancer. It was such a loss as she was a vibrant, beautiful, and a caring person and teacher. She and I met through our school district. Mary, also diagnosed with cancer, was an enthusiastic, dedicated, and expert teacher, and I was her principal. Through many years we shared stories of visiting our oncologists, treatments, and hair loss, and once a month we ate out at our favorite restaurant, enjoying dinner and one glass of wine that we allowed ourselves. Usually, it was on a Thursday night because that's the day she felt her best after a treatment.

Over 30 years our families got to know one another. Our children went to the same schools and we all went to the same church. When Mary retired from teaching, I even held her retirement party at my home. Since my husband was gone, my father who was living with me, helped as a co-host with Mary's husband, Chuck. The party was wonderful, joyous and the testimonials for Mary were numerous, heartfelt, and loving. In our retirements we continued our friendship with dinners, a cruise from New York to Canada, and frequent get-togethers. Sadly, four years after her retirement, Mary passed away. I was asked by the family to deliver her eulogy and I did so.

Now, fast forward a few months after Mary's passing to our retired-teachers-and-administrators discussion group at the local coffee house. In came Chuck, distressed and harried, stating, "I can't stay for long. My house is flooded from a cracked toilet, and I have a mess on my hands. Do you know someone I can call?"

I responded, "Call my son, Bill, a contractor. If he is free, he will help you." With the telephone number in hand, he raced from the coffee shop and, I found out later, that Bill had indeed come to his rescue.

Bill and Chuck worked all day, removed carpeting, cleaned up, drove to Home Depot for a new toilet, installed it, and finally finished around midnight. When they completed the project, Chuck paid Bill for his time and because he was so grateful asked him if there was anything he could do for him or his mother.

Bill answered much to Chuck's surprise, "Well, maybe you can take my Mom out to dinner." The next day when Bill told me what he said, I couldn't believe it.

He said, "It just popped out of my mouth, Mom, and I hope I didn't say the wrong thing."

I responded in complete shock, "What have you done?"

But almost immediately, Chuck called me and I accepted his invitation to dinner. I have to admit for a while it was a strange, awkward evening. Prior to this time, neither one of us had ever had a problem carrying on a conversation, but now the circumstances were different. We struggled a bit with inane questions and answers, but soon found that we had many common interests, values, and goals and had lots to talk about.

By the end of the evening, he asked if, at the end of the month, he could host a birthday dinner for me and invite some mutual friends. Surprised, happy, and caught short on words, I agreed, "Yes, that would be very nice."

That evening led to the birthday party, followed by a walk and lunch at the Arcadia Arboretum, a Chamber of Commerce luncheon, a meeting and lunch with my cousin, Carol, and soon after, a trip to Las Vegas. By Christmas time, we appeared nervously as a couple at a family celebration and a friend's Christmas party.

We speculated, "What will people say? Two old-timers dating?" And that was the beginning of the "gift" and our love story. Neither one of us realized that a plumbing disaster and a son's suggestion to "take my Mom to dinner" would bring us together and, eventually, lo and behold, after a year led us to the altar.

And here is the moral of my story of Blessings and a Gift:

Do not be afraid of opportunity. Take a chance, and listen to your heart. There may be a plan for you, something you have never thought possible or ever expected.

Cancer took my husband Bill and Chuck's wife Mary, but cancer also brought us together.

We don't think about how much time we will have and we don't dwell on the fact that cancer is a reoccurring factor in our lives. We deal with re-occurrences the best we can and continue to plan and enjoy trips, friends, get-togethers, and family good times. However, we feel blessed that we have the gift of love and we feel blessed that life gave us this time together.

— **Dr. Lois W. Neil**

Diagnosed with myeloproliferative disorder, a form of leukemia, Ela received a bone marrow transplant in July 2005. A teacher in the public schools of Los Angeles, she imparts knowledge to fourth and fifth grade

students, giving them positive perspectives on life. But, on one special day in a hospital hallway, Ela learned a life-changing lesson from a small child who never uttered a word.

Through a Child's Eyes

I was in my fourth week in Room 6211 in the Bone Marrow Transplant Unit at City of Hope, getting increasingly depressed and stuck in a crying jag. Everything made me cry. Despite daily visits from doctors, specialists, nurses, technicians, cafeteria staff, and family who were looking out for my health and well being, I couldn't shake the black mood I was spiraling into and going down fast.

Dr. Nakamura wrote a referral to the Psychiatric Department for an initial visit. A Ph.D. from Seattle doing a summer internship was assigned to my case. Young, still wet behind the ears, tall, and about 26 years old, he was half my age.

I knew he still had a lot to learn and still needed to pay his dues, so I did a quick study of his psychiatric game and answered all of his questions, gave all the right answers, made all the appropriate gestures and body movements. I was aware of his studying observations of me while he wrote his case notes. I also knew immediately that this path wasn't the "quick fix" I was looking for.

I wanted to jump out of this depression and I wanted to do it fast — like yesterday. I knew intellectually what was happening, but I felt I had no control.

I felt helpless and continued to look for an answer.

It came on a Thursday, three days later.

As I attempted a short walk in the hallway outside my room, I spotted a small Red Flyer wagon heading my way. It was being pulled by two female nurses. Sitting in the wagon was a two-year-old girl, surrounded by blankets, pillows, balloons, and stuffed animals. Like me, she had received a bone marrow transplant.

As we approached one another, I saw she was bald and her red cheeks were swollen and as big as a chipmunk's. In a split second, we looked at one another.

I had never seen a cancer baby. She was my first. As our eyes met, she started to laugh and point at me. I guess she liked the fact that we both were bald. But what she did next gave me the answer I had been seeking.

She tugged at a yellow balloon tied to her small wrist and offered it to me. I was at a loss for words.

Stunned, I pointed back to myself, "For me?"

She laughed her response, nodding her head. I looked at one of her nurses for confirmation and she also nodded.

I took the balloon and wanted to hug the tiny child, but I couldn't take the chance. We were both guarded with masks and gloves.

My answer came in what I saw in her eyes. I saw my rebirth. I saw hers. I saw that she and I were the same, struggling to live in the present, looking forward to a new life.

We were both dealt the cancer cards and we chose to deal life back into them. It didn't matter her age or mine; we were both the same. I saw that life could still have laughter and potential. She had both, why couldn't I?

As the nurses continued to pull her down the hallway in the wagon, I returned to my room and saw a different view outside my window. Instead of the dark and ominous San Gabriel Mountains looming in the distance, I could see the rocky path I needed to climb to the top of the mountain.

— **Ela Cabral**

In class, Robin, who loves rodeo, travels cross country with her friend Bubba in his 18-wheeler and faces adversity head-on, explains the gift of learning she had myelodysplasia, an incurable disease.

"Live Like You're Dying"

I hope you get the chance to live like you're dying. No, really, think about it. I found that although painful as it is, it seems as if there are only a handful of us, a select few, who have received this gift.

Yeah, right, you might say. Tim McGraw's song isn't for you?

When you think you're dying, it's time to learn just how precious life is and how fast it can be changed forever. When I was diagnosed, I decided what was, and is, important in life. I learned who I wanted to spend time with and who I could live without, who was friend and who was foe. Sometimes I question why God has put me on this path.

I even have days when I question whose moccasins I'm walking in.

But living with a life-threatening illness has been like riding a rodeo bull named Fu Man Chu, only the eight seconds doesn't come all that fast.

When the doctors told me that I had myelodysplasia with anemia and that there was no cure, I was devastated. I remember crying for what seemed like two straight months. It took time for me to realize that through this process, I had been given the gift of my mom, my brother, and my relatives. It has taken a lot of work, time, and forgiveness to get where we all needed to be.

Today, my illness is behaving and I am adjusting to also being a diabetic, but my life is sweet, if you'll pardon the pun. I have days when I'm still riding that same bull named Fu Man Chu. It's just that the eight seconds goes by a whole lot faster now.

So, tell me, how's your ride?

— **Robin Clarke**

(After writing this, Robin was hospitalized for 10 days. Upon arriving home, she spent her time in recovery making two quilts for fellow cancer patients and starting a Quilting for Life group.)

When asked to write about a gift he treasured most in life, Rick had no trouble.

Best Gift Ever

The best gift I ever received was the survival of my oldest son, Rick. I believed that God graced me with an awakening one day that everything was going to be okay with my son's treatment. The mantel of darkness, which had haunted me for months, was lifted from my being.

I walked differently, viewed the world euphorically, saw birds and heard music once again, where before I had seen stop lights and listened to traffic. I was almost giddy when I visited my son that afternoon, yet didn't tell him of my gift. He saw it and felt it, from my manner, and I'm certain shared in it somehow.

Now I still do much the same as I've always done, attend church only occasionally, and criticize when I feel strongly.

But now I believe that the heaviest drag on my soul was released by a God I had called upon in the darkest period of my journey.

— Rick Myers

As she read, Joy's description of her unforgettable "gift" made the class laugh out loud. It might have been her tone of voice, her smile, her cynical words, or the combination. Although legally blind, we often agree that Joy can "see" better than any of us. Her unwanted gift came when

someone disappeared from her life. By the time she finished reading, the class was no longer laughing. Instead, they were inspired.

Virtual Body Bag

They say good things come in small packages, but this was big! A monstrosity! A great big "body bag" was shoved in my face. It created such panic within me that I could not touch or examine it for some time. The deliverer of this ominous package, the one who almost wrecked my emotional seismograph, presented it with a speech that went like this:

"I will never be the person you want me to be. You are a good woman with a lot of gifts. You will do better without me. Head for the sun."

"So you're choosing the darkness then?" was my shocked response.

For the next three months, working around this bag, this symbol of death, so suddenly projected into the center of my existence, I ran myself ragged. It was my effort to evade the inevitable.

I discarded old furniture and junk. I cleaned and cleaned. I haggled with the landlord for a fresh coat of paint and new carpet. I needed to do anything but contemplate the contents of the dreaded bag. Still, there is sat.

When there was nothing else to clean, I left to spend time out of state with my family. There was no escaping, however, because I had to return home and confront my new reality.

I knew it was finally time to delve into my unwelcome gift. As I unzipped the body bag and began removing its packaging, I realized why I had been so afraid of this task.

Piece by piece I pulled out the excess baggage: anger, resentment, insecurity, guilt, blame, shame, and failure. There was also such an abundance of pain and fear inside that I had to stop.

The following day, I continued my task of completely emptying this strange gift bag, certain that I would not welcome its contents. For weeks I continued unearthing more conflict, pain, and tears, still not finding anything of value. By now, several friends had told me that I looked as if a load had been lifted off my shoulders. I thought they were crazy, just trying to make me feel good. I felt like crawling into that bag and zipping it around me. But there was so much left inside that I painfully continued to empty its contents.

Then suddenly one morning, digging deeper than I had gone before, I grasped something firm between my fingers. Unwrapping it cautiously, I found new enlightenment. I was stunned. There in my hand was a jewel whose brilliance beckoned to the rays of sunlight that were streaming in through my windows.

Suddenly surrounded by all that light, I knew that there in my hand I held my personal freedom. I was momentarily bewildered. How could this be? My broken heart was real. My pain was real. This treasure in my hand was also real. What would I do with it?

Among the wretchedness of the excess baggage left for me by my fleeing spouse was a gift, a pearl of incomparable value. I was free! Free even to grant myself the time and space needed to mend my broken heart, free to grieve my losses without taunting or degradation. I was free to recognize how, in weakness, I had not sufficiently valued this gem.

Incidentally, the day my body bag was delivered, I had also given a gift. I presented my departing spouse with a book called *Healing for the Masculine Soul*.

I don't know if he ever opened his gift, but I had opened mine and life has been good ever since.

— Joy E. Walker Steward

Abigail, 15, a sophomore at Bonita High School, La Verne, California, admitted being reluctant when she volunteered to help cancer patients for eight hours. Her initial motivation was to fill the square of "community service" on her college application forms. Instead, it became a life-changing day.

Stacey's Gift

I drummed my fingers on the armrest of the car. My wristwatch read 8:30. Hmmm, I thought, that means I have about seven and a half hours to volunteer, a small dent in the amount I need to get into a good college, but it's a start. My mom pulled up in front of the City of Hope's Pediatric Bone Marrow Transplant Cancer Unit. I sighed. This is not how I want to spend my day. But, oh well, here goes nothing.

When I arrived inside the building, the head nurse directed me to a patient's room on the right side of the wing.

She turned to me, "This little girl's name is Stacey, she's two years old, and you'll be watching her today. Her mom has not left her side for the past two months, and she wants to run a few errands. Just press the nurse's call button if you need help."

Great. This is not exactly what I thought I'd be doing as a volunteer, now I am dealing with a living, breathing child.

After putting on a surgical mask, I carefully opened the door of the hospital room. As my eyes adjusted to the dim light, I could barely make out the figure of a bald little girl lying in bed, surrounded by coloring books and crayons on one side and dolls and stuffed animals on the other.

The television was on. More gifts lined the walls, some opened and others still wrapped. A woman who seemed to be the girl's mother poked her head out of the adjoining bathroom. She was in the process of curling her long brown hair.

"Hi! You must be Abby. I'm just going to finish getting ready and I'll be back about 2:30."

As I responded with a simple, "Great," my eyes continued scanning the room.

She must be living in this room; it looks like she doesn't leave often.

Her bags and clothes were scattered about the room, making it look cramped and uncomfortable.

After she left, I attempted to keep Stacey occupied by helping her color and play her favorite programs on television. I also learned that Stacey's diaper had to be changed every 30 to 45 minutes. This procedure was nothing like what I faced in my previous babysitting experiences.

The process required two nurses and me to change Stacey's diaper, her bed sheets, and her blankets. Just picking her up wreaked havoc on her frail little body, and she responded with screams that rang down the hall. Something in Stacey's cancer medication caused her to experience severe pain, making her feel as if she were covered with bruises from head to toe.

All I could do was hold her and rock her gently back and forth, but even that just made her wail louder. Every time we began to change her, Stacey would turn her face towards me and glare as if I had personally betrayed her. My function as the playful, fun babysitter was gone, and my role as torturer had commenced. It broke my heart that I could do nothing to ease her pain.

She's so young. She doesn't even know that we are trying to help her or that our actions are for her own good. This medicine will hopefully save her life.

It struck me how this same scenario occurred in my relationship with God when I had suffered losses.

When people I loved hurt me, I would scream at God, "This is not fair!" I would look around at my fallen world and doubt God. Why would

He cause pain, let such horrible things happen to me, things I didn't deserve? I would feel betrayed.

Just as Stacey was looking into my compassionate yet knowing face, I looked into the eyes of a loving God who realized the reasons why I had to go through such tribulations. Through these hardships and trials, He was refining my character so I could serve Him better.

After a while Stacey became restless and lost interest with her available means of entertainment. She cried constantly for her mother, probably because she had never been left alone for more than a few minutes at a time.

All I could try was to comfort her and try to keep her attention diverted by playing with dolls and coloring, but to no avail. Finally, one of the nurses suggested that I put Stacey into a little red wagon they kept on hand and pull her around the circular hospital's hallways. I propped Stacey up with some pillows and covered her with a blanket.

We started off, and I attempted to manage both the IV pole and the wagon with my two hands. After one full turn I looked back at her. She had not made a sound since we started, and now her tear-streaked face had turned peaceful as she looked out curiously at everything we passed by. I smiled.

Finally I had figured out something to make her feel better. This seemed to do the trick.

To keep Stacey from erupting into sobs again, I walked her around that circular hospital wing twenty or thirty times. How odd we must have looked. But instead of causing me to feel embarrassed, this motion provided me with a growing sense of joy. For the first time all day I was providing something soothing for her, not just something she needed, but something that she really wanted, something she couldn't do for herself.

Stacey sat content, enjoying this small, feeble gift I had to offer her. My feet walked the familiar path, and I became lost in my own thoughts.

During the course of that day, my motive for being there began to change. Instead of looking to merely boost my involvement in community activities for college, I began to focus my efforts on providing the best help to Stacey that I could.

I learned how to schedule my actions to her agenda, her comfort being foremost on my mind.

I was shocked by how easy it became for me to adopt this kind of mindset with Stacey, yet I still lacked this level of dedication to God. Stacey's situation caused me to look at my life from a different perspective. I can now see that God has given me so much, my health, my family, my friends, my life — things dangerously fluctuating, tentative, and even missing entirely in young Stacey's life.

I believe that God used this experience to correct my attitude. I came to volunteer that day with the self-righteous idea that I was sacrificing my valuable time; I was under the impression that I was providing this great service to the hospital.

One sick little girl taught me to treasure things, to see God in everything, a gift that remains priceless to this day, worth more than anything I could have hoped to give her, and worth so much more than the number of volunteer hours written on any college application.

— Abigail Palmer

Nina is a mother, a teacher, and the daughter of a cancer survivor. Little did she know that she and her hound dog would share common medical problems and outcomes.

Lucky in Cancer — Me and My Dog

Nine years ago I had my first diagnosis of breast cancer; four years later it had metastasized to my liver. I was lucky. It has responded to minimal treatment (hormonal), and all traces have been gone from the dreaded PET scan for five years.

What has changed for me is that I can't help being cheerful. I awake each day knowing that cancer has been, and is part of my life; but I'm okay at the moment. More than okay. I'm healthy and cheerful and energized. I now have more "moments" ahead of me. I just can't find it in myself to be depressed.

I also sing with my Sweet Adeline sisters and enjoy the relaxation that comes from breathing and moving to music. I can't help but find the positive in most activities I do and people I meet.

While they say animals tend to resemble their owners, my dog and I started to have similar medical illnesses. My hound dog, Ozark, had a large cancerous tumor removed from his side four years ago. A year ago another cancerous tumor appeared, but this time he also had tumors in his lungs.

I decided "no surgery" because we were going to lose him soon; the vet had said six to eight weeks. That was one year ago and soon he is going to celebrate his 14th birthday. We finally did the surgery and he is still his happy, tail-wagging, cheerful, naughty self with cancer that has stopped growing.

We both have experienced cancer. We are both lucky. We are both cheerful at the moment.

There must be a country-western song here.

— **Nina Steinberg**

Donna came to class only once. The day's assignment was to write about a special gift. She told the group that she viewed her most valued gift in life as the opportunity she had to serve as the caregiver for her friend who was dying from breast cancer. She read her poem aloud.

The Exchange

A woman's breast is the cradle for the weary soul.
And in your grief I would hold you,
Tarry until peace was exchanged for peace, spirit for spirit,
In the place where comfort comes from the omnipotent source,
Tender circling arms, the place of the rendering.
And when your emptiness filled,
And the salt of your tears was but a blanket upon your skin,
Then I would linger, holding you a bit longer,
And closer, and more dear.
For my need to give was as great as yours in the taking.
So the gift was ours,
An exchange of two weary souls in need.

— Donna Lee Holland

The day she returned home from the hospital after a week of intense chemotherapy in preparation for her first bone marrow transplant, Christine saw life itself as a gift.

How Blessed I Am

Life is not achieving material success, fame, or fortune. Life is growing, sharing, and living fully each splendid, delicious moment. It is a gift to experience this life in a physical body. The meaning of life is to make this world a better place for others and for the future.

Dear God, give me complete healing so that I may continue to share and celebrate this gift.

While in this world, live fully. All the love you give is the joy you will feel when it is finally time for you to pass over. It is love that brings the tears of thanks for a life well lived. It is love that makes the crux of your core, that feeds you, that gives you strength in softness. It is the binding force of this universe. It makes us compassionate souls. It gives us the ability to look beyond ourselves and see the beauty and poetry of this world.

The illness taught me how precious each moment is, how beautiful this life is, and how blessed I am.

— Christine Pechera

It's Your Turn

What has having a life-threatening disease or experiencing a tragedy brought you or taught you? Express your feelings in as much detail as possible. Remember gifts can be given or received. What is the greatest gift you have received? What is the greatest gift you have ever given? Use the sentences below if you need help getting started.

Jump Start

Through this (tragedy, diagnosis, treatment) my most cherished gift is ...

A gift I would like to give or have given someone else is ...

Chapter 15

Choosing Happiness

If a smile from a stranger could move me, I'd invite it in.

— Robin Clarke

After much planning for a weekend getaway, my husband and I find ourselves in Albuquerque at its annual "Balloon Fiesta" in October.

Onlookers by the thousands start arriving at 5 a.m., wending their way into the parking lots that surround the grassy 55-acre site. We have heard about the event for years and know that participants come from all over the world.

Dressed in jackets, gloves, hats, and warm pants, newcomers like us Californians not used to cold weather begin to doubt if the sun will ever come up. We can still see the stars. We can also see our breath! Will we get frostbite?

When we arrive, none of the balloons have been inflated. Hundreds of people mill around, blowing on their hands to keep warm and buying breakfast burritos from the vendors.

168

Then the "Dawn Patrol" goes up. Two massive balloons are quickly inflated and are sent aloft to test the winds — to see if conditions are safe for the hundreds of others waiting patiently on the ground. If the winds are too strong, the remaining balloons will be grounded, but if winds are favorable, all the others will get the okay to "fly."

Just seeing those first two is thrilling. They start to rise as silhouetted shapes only. When they get about 25 feet into the air, the gas burners turn on in hissing spurts and the huge teardrops glow with color. Then they become silent silhouettes again. Conditions are judged favorable and the news is radioed back to the ground where it is broadcast to the crowd. The waiting crews have the okay to fly. Spectators cheer and clap. Tension builds.

A few minutes later, still in the pitch-black cold, crew members start to remove the huge balloons from their vehicles and prepare them for inflation. Everywhere we look, large wicker baskets are being taken from the backs of pickup trucks and vans. Massive bundles of cloth are laid out on the grass. We try to stay warm by drinking hot chocolate and coffee from vendors and soon we forget about the cold as we watch the first act of a unique ballet. Dawn has begun to lift the night's curtain.

The performance has started, but the dancers still have their feet on the ground.

Next to us stands a team of eight, all dressed in hot pink outfits and wearing matching pink cowboy hats. They are clearly excited but also obviously skilled. Each person has a job to do.

At their leader's signal, they begin pulling and straightening a massive piece of hot pink material. In a few minutes, with the help of a huge fan and lots of crew members and even some spectators who hold the basket upright and steady the balloon with tether ropes, it begins to rise.

Before our eyes, in just a few minutes, it grows into what looks like a ten-story-high hot-pink elephant, complete with trunk curved and pointed skyward in a victory salute.

Who could not delight in this? Children and adults alike utter loud sighs and then cheer as the massive elephant takes to the skies.

Words really cannot describe what 700 colorful hot-air balloons look like as they rise en masse at dawn over the New Mexico landscape. The sky becomes a painting. It is thrilling beyond belief.

And it costs only $5 to park and $5 for admission, cheaper than a ticket to a bad movie.

Following the "mass assent" of 700 regular hot-air balloons, the 89 "shapes" of everything from a Space Shuttle replica, a balloon actually larger than the Shuttle itself, to a 16-story-high green dragon rise gracefully.

Soon the crowd thins out as the day's main attractions begin to drift off in the wind, becoming mere dots on the horizon.

We decide to leave the balloon site and take an aerial tram ride up to the top of Sandia Mountain, part of a large and rocky backdrop overlooking the entire area. We hope to see the balloons again from up there. Our spirits are high and the day holds great promise as we drive to the base of the mountain.

We get in line for the tram tickets, still scanning the skies for glimpses of the wind riders.

Behind us in line is a middle-aged woman who apparently hasn't seen what we just have. She is frowning and her tone of voice is harsh.

"I can't believe those people are just cutting in line!" she barks, pointing to some senior citizens, apparently on a group tour, who pass us and head directly for the tram.

A closer look would have revealed they all held tickets in their hands, probably already bought and paid for as part of their package deal.

"This is ridiculous!" she says again, trying to get the rest of us in line to agree to mutiny, to riot — who knows?

Next, she unloads on the two women who are with her, this time about another subject.

"You know I'm just going to have to sue our gardener!" she says, loud enough so we all know she is rich enough to have one. "He dumped dirt on our tennis court — not the clay court, mind you, the hard-surface one — and, well, he ruined it!"

The other women kind of grunt. They have obviously been with her a long time.

"I'm sick, I tell you, sick over it!"

More grunts.

We stand in line for about 20 minutes, listening to her litany of complaints about the money her physician husband has to pay for his insurance, the fact that the building they own is too small to expand his practice, and, well, you get the idea.

There we are in one of the most beautiful spots in the country with hundreds of other enthusiastic tourists determined to enjoy ourselves, and this angry woman is ruining our day.

Bob leans over to me and whispers in my ear, "God I'm glad I'm not married to her!" He kisses me on the cheek. We both laugh and decide without any more words that she isn't going to ruin our day or even another minute of it. We begin to laugh each time she complains about something new.

We have tuned out her venom. We have, in effect, chosen happiness.

Many of us can probably recall similar situations when people try to rain on our parade. It becomes our choice as to whether we let the day be ruined.

But, having cancer or another serious illness isn't something you can just tune out, ignore, and go about your business. What you can do, though, is limit the effect that negative people and negative events have on your life.

Over a period of several months, I had surgery five times. One of my saline breast implants went flat and the doctor said I needed to have both replaced because they only last about seven years. It had been seven years, almost to the day. Funny how those warranty things work. After the surgeries, I had staph infections twice and had to return to the operating table. I didn't sing and dance my way out and back to the hospital, but I did make a conscious decision to put the negatives into the proper perspective.

In between those trips to the doctor and the hospital, I chose to go to the Balloon Fiesta, to hike in the Canadian Rockies, and to attend a symphony concert or two in California. I also chose to leave the local hospital where my first surgeries took place and go to the City of Hope where they routinely perform cancer reconstruction surgeries.

Ultimately, I had a bi-lateral "tram-flap" operation, ending forever the need for future breast implants and flattening my tummy at the same time. A nice tradeoff. Thank you, Dr. James Andersen for the 12 hours of microsurgery and all the training you received and now provide to other doctors.

Healing Words

When I give students the assignment to write about choosing happiness, some interesting and varied writings result from that lesson.

Students are in various stages of cancer treatment and recovery when they come to class. They often write about the "passages" they are going through.

The chapters in this book move from the shock of diagnosis through anger and into recovery, the same way as your attitudes toward the disease or tragedy and how you cope with them.

Your attitude as you recover is everything. You can choose to be that doctor's wife on top of the mountain, too angry to see anything beautiful or inspirational around you. Or you can choose to take your mind and, ultimately, your body to positive venues. You have a choice.

Instead of watching the evening news with its predictable negatives, renting a video of a romantic comedy may be your choice. It may also be a better prescription for your wellness.

Joan's title is her statement about how she lives her life.

I Choose Happiness

My friend, Mary, was diagnosed with breast cancer five years ago, just shortly after I was diagnosed. If you meet Mary today, though, she'll tell you, "I HAVE breast cancer."

She had a lumpectomy, radiation, and chemotherapy. Tamoxifen makes her sick, but she won't speak to her doctor about making a change in her medication. She has little pleasure in living because she has chosen to be a cancer patient for the rest of her life.

I had a mastectomy, radiation, and chemotherapy. I chose to believe I would recover, mostly because the opposite choice was too scary for me to contemplate.

When I talk about it, I always say, "I HAD breast cancer."

That is what I believe.

I wake up every morning, or at least most mornings, glad to be alive. I brew a cup of coffee and sit by the window in my new apartment, watching the sailboats set out for the day.

Some days I read the newspaper and do the crossword puzzle. Sometimes I go for a walk beside the ocean, or visit a friend, either in person or on the phone.

There is laundry to do, shopping, perhaps or dishes, or dusting. They will wait.

I choose to do the things that make me happy as often as I can.

That's not to say that I never have a bad day. But when I do, I try to remember that I have a choice.

Cancer has taught me a lesson I hope never to forget.

— Joan Smith

Edna's choice came early in her life. She was in college when her mother died from leukemia. Her relationship with her father was strained. Her decision to move out and on has made all the difference.

The Fork in the Road

When I think about my choices after my mother died, there weren't a lot of them: stay with my father at home or move out. Neither was good.

I had no idea how I would support myself, and I needed the security of familiar surroundings. But, if I stayed, I would have him to deal with.

Go or stay?

Through my incredible grief, pain, loss, and despair, the answer was far from clear. Separate or remain joined? Daughter or surrogate wife? Compliant or defiant?

I chose happiness.

You do what you can do, one day at a time.

— Edna Teller

Her daughter, Donna, a young mother of three, had just been told she had breast cancer for the third time. Theda could have wallowed in her own pain and sorrow. Instead she wrote about a special and symbolic gift from her daughter.

The Fuchsia

Donna gave me an old-time sieve used for making jelly. I loved it. It was a long time before I planted anything in it but then one day I did and I hung it on the front porch.

Fuchsias have been one of my favorite plants; their pretty little bell-like flowers fascinate me. Their common name is "bleeding heart."

I had planted fuchsias before, but they died. But, when I planted this fuchsia in the antique sieve, I did so with determination. This time it was a symbol of my daughter's life. It would not fail.

As it grew, I watered it diligently, reveled in its blooms, sure that this was the omen I needed.

She would be all right, just like the plant. She would bloom and survive.

I was sure it wasn't the proper vessel for perfect growth, but it began growing and blooming. The challenge must be met.

Donna found another lump. This wasn't in the plan. The omen may have failed me.

I continued to water, nourish, and love the plant. It's still an omen.

It is still alive. So is she.

— Theda Clark

In Dave Key's Do-It newsletter sent to his friends and family as he struggled to survive, he has a cartoon with two women chatting over the garden fence.

One says to the other, "Have a nice day!"
The other responds, "I always decide to make it a nice day."
It is a choice, Dave reminds us.

Christine, recovering from her first bone marrow transplant, watches with new eyes the spectacular waterfall on the hospital grounds, a waterfall that at one time gave her pause.

Spring

The waterfall today does not remind me of a hundred thousand tears.
But reminds me of life and its infinite source.
It does not remind me of suffering.
But gives me quiet hope.
I do not hear the cries of cancer victims in the falling water,
But the joys and shouts of survivors singing.
The sound of the water does not make me cry; it fills me.
And those who have passed on do not mourn for their lives,
But lovingly smile down, blessings from heaven.

— Christine Pechera

Whenever Janet is in class, she exudes a calmness, an acceptance of others, a sense of kindness that is completely natural. Clearly, she has already chosen happiness.

Angel Wings

Wouldn't it be something to fly on angels' wings?
To float on top of clouds and see so many beautiful things?
Softly and gently, along as we go,
Floating and drifting over the rainbow?
To pull up the sunrise and lay down the sunset,

To see such beauty we should never forget?
Oh wouldn't it be something to fly on angels' wings,
To feel the peace and contentment of all glorious things?

— Janet Gray

Their motto, "There's Always Hope," is seen throughout the City of Hope. Anna, recovering from colon cancer, dedicated the following poem to just-diagnosed cancer patients she encounters as a volunteer, escorting them to appointments, treatments, and laboratories. Her poem was printed in the campus newsletter Hope *Notes.*

Hope

I see the look upon your face,
Longing for a warm embrace.
I see the tears flow down your cheeks,
It's not a sign that you are weak.
I know your fear, for I've been there.
I want you to know that I do care.
I will be near to help you cope,
And remind you "There is always hope."

— Anna Andrizzi Escobosa

Even a winter windstorm in California is seen as positive by Robert.

The Sea of Wind

Wind is blowing very hard on this December day. Winds are coming over and through the mountains with a thunderous roar.

You can hear and see it through the trees far away, bending closer and
closer like mighty waves breaking at the seashore.

The palm trees bend like crescent moons.

The leaves of the trees swirl all around the yard.

The leaves start to build up at the fence, just like a wave at the beach.

What a thought — my own personal wave!

How beautiful to see the tops of the trees bending and swaying and their
trunks standing firm and strong.

Just like us bending with our problems with our feet firmly on the
ground.

I feel like I'm lost on my own tropical island, inside this sea of wind, not
wanting to be found.

Surely, I'm in heaven while still alive.

— Robert Prado

It's Your Turn

You've heard the advice to make lemonade out of the lemons life
gives us. You've also heard about the half-full, half-empty optimism test.
Both are examples of the same theory: you are in charge. You can see
your illness as a tragedy, the end of life, and live each day accordingly.
Or, you can choose hope and happiness like Joan, Edna, Theda,
Christine, Anna, and Robert. You decide.

Write about a time in your life when you were faced with such a
choice. Perhaps you are going through that process at this time. How are
you dealing with it? Do you surround yourself with people who choose
happiness? Has cancer or a tragedy changed the choices you are making?

Jump Start

I made a conscious decision to choose happiness when ...

When something negative happens, I find myself ...

Describe the effect reading and writing about this subject had on you.

Chapter 16

Laughter as Medicine

What are the three little words every woman wants to hear from her man?
"I was wrong!"

— Charlton Heston

Living so close to Hollywood, it is not uncommon to be able to see famous actors appearing in stage productions or giving speeches at charity events. I went to a political fundraiser where Charlton Heston gave his oration on "The Death of Moses" and, as I expected, it was inspirational and spellbinding. He spoke from memory for about 20 minutes, his booming voice captivating the crowd. Nobody in the place moved for several seconds after he finished. Even those who don't agree with his politics had tears in their eyes.

Just prior to that, though, he had warmed up the crowd with the above quote. He said somebody asked him how he stayed married to the same woman for decades, a rarity in Hollywood.

He told the crowd he had advice to give the men in the audience and, if they listened, they would learn something. Then he told them about those three little words and he brought down the house.

Whenever I have repeated his advice, people laugh out loud. A good laugh is always welcome, but especially when going through the trials of medical treatments.

You have probably heard the saying, "If I didn't laugh, I'd cry."

Doctors and operating room personnel will tell their friends, off the record, that many times at the height of a difficult surgery, someone in the operating room will crack a joke. Many times they aren't about medicine, either.

Students in Writing for Wellness class are told to think of a memory that always makes them laugh. It does not have to relate to cancer or anything medical. When students recall a vivid memory, it often involves being embarrassed, trying to be someone other than yourself, or doing something you shouldn't and getting caught in the act.

I give them two examples from my life.

I always had bad eyes. I wore glasses in the sixth grade.

By the time I was in high school, I had contact lenses, but those were the old hard style that made your eyes flood with tears and your eyelids turn pink as you blinked continuously.

More often than not, I chose to wear no glasses or contacts. In typical teenage logic, I thought they made me look ugly. And I never, ever wore them on dates, for heaven's sake. The fact that the world looked completely blurry to me was a side effect I accepted.

One night, a new young man in my high school class asked me to go out. His idea of a date was to go to the miniature golf course in Manitou Springs, about 10 miles from my house in Colorado Springs. This meant an older friend of his would have to drive us. It was a double date.

I didn't golf well, even with glasses. Without them, I was hopeless.

Half way through the game, I hit the ball too hard and it bounced up and over into another "fairway" almost out of sight. As I was looking to see where my ball landed, I stepped forward and fell flat into a water hazard that was about three feet deep. I got soaked and I made a lasting impression on the new boy in town.

Funny, he never called me again.

The scene repeated itself after I got married and my husband was an Air Force pilot. We had been invited to his commanding officer's home for a cocktail party. I was excited and spent the afternoon getting my hair done, polishing my fingernails, and selecting just the right outfit. The entire squadron's pilots and spouses had been invited.

Of course, I decided to not wear my glasses.

We seemed to be the last to arrive, passing cars parked bumper-to-bumper along the curb near his house. Finding a space, we hurried to his door. Just as we entered his home, he met us with some drinks, which he was serving from a tray.

I took a glass of wine and a step toward what I thought was a rather fuzzy living room with a nice flat floor. Instead, I fell down several stairs into his "sunken" room. And I made quite a splash. I also think I heard someone comment about my having a drinking problem.

Once I water skied without my glasses and couldn't see the boat, but that's a whole other story.

Healing Words

In class, as I describe some of my own disasters, students begin to smile, recall their own unforgettable moments, and start to write. Giggling fills the room and smirks come over their faces as the group records their memories on paper. After about 15 minutes, poems, songs, and slice-of-life essays emerge.

It was after one lesson on laughter when people in class realized, for the first time, that we had a celebrity in our midst. Class members knew Elizabeth only as a patient battling an especially aggressive breast cancer. We had seen her without hair and with bandages on her arms. We all knew she was from England and had a delightful style and accent when she read her words aloud. She had written about her own battles. She had briefly mentioned that she was a professional writer but had not gone into specifics. She had also agreed to substitute teach for me when I had surgery. Everyone in class knew her and liked her.

What they didn't know was that Elizabeth was known to the world outside the classroom as someone who had written news stories about Princess Diana nearly every week for four years. She had also been personally invited to and had attended Diana's funeral in Westminster Abbey. She revealed this as a preface for what she had just finished writing.

As she started to read, we all wondered, what could possibly be funny about any of that?

My Bridget Jones Moment

It all started innocently enough. The usual dinner-party banter. But this was in August in New York, the Hamptons, with a media-heavy group of journalists and television producers, friends of the friends we were staying with.

When the subject came to Princess Diana, the anniversary of her death was fast approaching, our hostess said, "Oh, Elizabeth can tell you everything about Di; she wrote about her every week for four years while working in London for *People* and *In Style.*"

So the questions began: what was she like, how did she talk, was she really a little crazy, the funeral — how was it being inside the Abbey, what was the atmosphere like, who else did you see there, the princes — were they crying? And Charles, how did he behave?

The evening ended and my husband and I left the Hamptons a couple of days later to spend time in New York City before heading back to Los Angeles.

Early one morning at the hotel, the phone rang, "Hi Elizabeth. This is Bruce. I'm a producer at CNN. I met you at Charla's dinner party at Sag Harbor the other night. Hey, I thought it would be fun for you to be a panelist on a show we're doing about Princess Diana's legacy on the anniversary of her death this Friday."

Fun? I liked the way he phrased that.

I insisted that I was not the expert he was looking for and he countered that I was just perfect, articulate for television and full of good anecdotes of what the Princess was really like and how tragic her death was.

"It'll be just like you were talking at the dinner — very easy and low key."

By Friday when I got back to LA in the early morning, I had really forgotten having sort of agreed to the assignment. No one had called me regarding the details so I figured it was not happening.

What a wrong assumption that was.

Then the phone rang. A producer was calling to say a car would be picking me up at 1 p.m. to take me to the CNN studios in Hollywood.

She didn't have any details for me on what the show was about, but she did mutter something about it being live. LIVE? I had done segments before for CNN, but they were always taped.

What kind of a show was this?

"Greta Van Susteren — to the Point," she responded matter-of-factly.

"Wasn't she that barking lawyer on television?" I asked myself.

"No more time for questions," said the producer. "Be ready at 1 p.m."

As I waited for the car, I felt I was being taken to my execution. How did innocent me get roped into this tortuous exercise? And they weren't even paying me.

When I arrived at the studio, I bumped into Larry King, which only made me feel worse. This really was happening at CNN, I suddenly realized.

The hair and makeup people greeted me and fixed me up, as they put it, and escorted me through to the "green room." I still just couldn't believe this was happening.

Soon I was summoned to another small room with a chair in front of the classic cheesy Hollywood background — the Hollywood sign on the Hollywood Hills and then there was that camera equipment with a camera operator whose gender I couldn't immediately recognize.

That was unnerving in and of itself and did nothing to calm me down.

"How do I look?" I asked meekly?

"FINE!" it answered. "Just look into the camera and speak. Don't start looking at the monitors on the side."

Then, in my earpiece, I heard a producer's voice from Atlanta and next Greta's barking voice from Washington.

"This is great! Bruce said you're just great! It's going to be a great show. Ready to roll."

I was steadily going into shock. First came the introductions of the panelists: *Time Magazine's* executive editor; the Washington correspondent for the BBC; Christopher Anderson, a noted biographer on the royals, and then little me: Elizabeth Terry, a royal contributor to *People*.

"No!" I screamed to myself.

I had already explained to the producer that they must introduce me as a freelance writer in Hollywood since my editor at *People* specifically did not want anyone associated with the magazine on that show.

What should I do? Correct Greta on air and have her beat me up mercilessly for the rest of the program or let it fly and have my editor berate me later?

I opted for the second choice but my eyes flashed pretty wildly from side to side as I tried to figure this one out.

Then came the barrage of questions from Miss Van Susteren: "Elizabeth, would you call Diana's death a global death?"

"What kind of nonsense abstract trick question is that?" I thought to myself. Wait a minute. I thought I was supposed to talk about Diana's sartorial dress sense, her charity work, and the atmosphere in Westminster Abbey at her funeral. I had all those details in my head. This was definitely turning into an out-of-body experience and I wasn't sure if I was going to cry or simply pass out.

But then, like a miracle sent down from the heavens, I suddenly learned the art of counter-punching Van Susteren's fiery, not-applicable-to-me questions with the finesse of a politician batting off nasty interviewers on news programs.

I just talked about what I knew and then, of course, it was time for the panelists to sign off. I slid off my chair as if I just been on the Revolution ride at Magic Mountain a hundred times.

I asked the camera operator, "How do you think it went?"

"Okay," pausing for an awkward moment, "but you might want to brush your hair before you leave the building."

What?

I looked in the mirror and my hair was a complete disaster, as if I had a curtain covering my face with spiky bits sticking up from my scalp.

No doubt while waiting in the green room for my execution, I had unconsciously pulled at my hair as panic set in. The result: I looked like a freak on national TV and no one had bothered to tell me.

Needless to say that was my first and last national television experience.

— **Elizabeth Terry**

When Robin's grandmother, Katie Whitten, died at age 77 and was cremated, no one guessed she'd go on a ride and just keep on truckin'.

Grandma Katie's Wanderlust

I met a trucker named Bubba, or Big Rob, as some called him, when I fell into his lap. We had been sitting on a couch talking and when I started to get up, my knees and hips went out from under me. I landed in his lap. You might say I fell for him. It has been eight years since that night. Bubba is as big as life and as gentle as a cub.

My Grandma, who everyone called Katie, always loved the big trucks, the 18-wheelers. Even before I met Bubba, I had made her a promise that after she died, I would see to it that she was taken on one final "run" and that we'd leave her out on the open road.

Katie loved to travel. All anybody had to say was, "Road trip?" and she'd be ready to go.

Grandpa had died before her, and he wanted to be scattered where he loved to fish. Even now when someone calls our house not knowing he has passed away, I will tell them, "He on a fishing trip."

But Katie told us she didn't want any part of that.

She died seven months before I met Bubba.

A family friend, Alan, spent a lot of time on the road for his job delivering artwork around the country, and he also spent a lot of time at Katie's house. She got into the habit of putting out a plate for him every time he was in town. She always loved hearing about where he'd driven and what he'd seen because she'd been a lot of places, too.

Alan ate anything Grandma put in front of him. Even when she tried out new recipes or cooked one of her "mystery" meals, he'd always clean his plate.

So, after Grandma died and was cremated, we asked Alan if he'd take half of her on one of his road trips. He agreed and so I bottled her up in two large plastic seasoning bottles and gave him one. Katie was off with Alan like Mrs. Dash.

How many grandmas do you know who have been from Maine to California? Alan fulfilled Katie's wish and came home without her. Since there was still plenty of Katie left to go around, we decided to take her on one last ride with me and my friend, the trucker named Bubba.

To this day, the thought of going on my first big-rig run with Katie on her very last one brings a smile to my heart and a chuckle to my soul, just knowing that she is now at rest and at "home" on the road where we released her.

Eventually we all just keep on truckin' down that highway of life, keeping in mind to remember those periodic brake checks along the way.

— Robin Clarke

One obviously bald patient wears a colorful knit cap embroidered with the words, "Quiet! Hair Growing!" As many cancer patients know, a bad hair day for someone with hair is different from one for those without it. Using the writing technique of repeating the first words in every line, Carole writes about hair.

Bad Hair Day

Waiting for a haircut,
Waiting for hair to grow,
   bad news: cancer and chemo.
Waiting for hair to fall out,
Waiting still for hair to grow,
   good news — blonde wig and sexy red,
Waiting's not so bad now.

— Carole Palmquist

Joy described to the writing class how, following her divorce, she found humor on February 14th when her friends were opening their pink, heart-shaped boxes of candy and their lacy Valentine cards. She learned that sometimes being left out is not all bad. There are things worse than being alone.

She grinned like a Cheshire cat as her hands glided over the Braille on her paper and her words came forth in her Jamaican accent in a slightly cynical tone. She was loving it.

So What I Have No Valentine?

No love romantic is in my life,
For I am nobody's wife.
Nobody's whispering in my ear,
Some lie about how much he cares.
No gifts with strings or traps attached,
No dangling carrot I'll never catch.
No deadly dance my love to prove,
No headstands one cold heart to move.
No wondering why he is so late,
Nor why my person he berates.
No circular talk to drain my brain.
No more migraines or chest pains.
No more groveling for what is mine,
From some stingy Valentine.
Joy and light are in my life,
Don't need to be nobody's wife.
The loving messages I hear,
All come from friends who are sincere.
Now I think and dream and feel,

And know my feelings are quite real.
My giftedness is in full view.
I do whatever I choose to do.
My hope is high, my heart is free,
God says I'm special, and I love me.
So what I have no Valentine?
Just look at how much else is mine!

— Joy E. Walker Steward

It's Your Turn

Think back to a humorous experience. When the family gets together, do you ever tell old stories? Write about one of them or another humorous event in your life.

It doesn't have to be material for "Saturday Night Live," which I've never thought is all that funny anyway. Just recalling the event may bring you a smile and warm your heart. Use the sentences below if you need a little help getting started.

Jump Start

I laugh out loud every time I think about the time when ...

I'll never forget the look on ...'s face when ...

Make an effort to recall those funny times when you find yourself stuck in traffic, waiting for a doctor's appointment, or just sitting at home feeling stressed or sad. You may get a smile when you least expect one.

Chapter 17

Mind-Mending Journeys

When my pain was so severe, so chronic, I would close my eyes and take myself to the mountain meadow in my mind.

— Christine Pechera

Where does your mind take you to mend? When life gets too complicated, when illness and negatives drag you down both physically and mentally, when hope seems far away, how do you cope?

Music works for many people. You put on your favorite music and, almost without knowing it, you may be singing along, tapping your foot, or totally swept away. Your mood changes and you are in another time and place. Whether it's western, jazz, rock, or classical, music can be your best and cheapest therapist.

You can also take down old photograph albums, dust them off, and flip though, thinking of better times and places and forcing your mind to mend from the days or weeks of treatments or check-ups, pre- and post-surgery visits and the pain of the most recent operation. Having a friend or family member with you can also be healing as the two of you journey back through wild and crazy days or wonderful and poignant ones.

After just a half an hour, your mind may be ready to resume its role in present reality.

Some of the best therapy for a weary mind, though, can involve writing. Getting cards and letters from our loved ones provides us with the comfort of knowing we aren't alone; somebody cares. Even a short note added to a commercial card can bring a smile. We prop up the cards near our bedsides and often save them long after we are well. It is hard to throw words away.

Telephone calls can also help us heal. Hearing a relative in another state cheer you on or getting a call from a high school or college friend who connects you with your past and, usually, simple and happy times, is always welcome.

But I read once that telephone calls can't be saved in a shoebox. That profound statement resonated with my students. We don't usually make recordings of telephone calls, although some people have actually saved voicemails informing them they got a job, a promotion, or an award. Most calls, even the good ones you would like to remember forever, disappear into thin air as the delete button is pushed.

If you want to make a lasting impact, write down your feelings.

Often in class students will be reading one of their writings, choke up, and have to stop. "I'm sorry," they always say.

My response is, "Never apologize for having emotions, only for *not* having them."

One assignment in Writing for Wellness is for students to answer the question, "Where does your mind take you to heal?"

Students tell me that when they write and consciously force their minds to go to another place, a place of comfort and healing, something wonderful happens. They are surprised how much it helps them escape from their present-day pains when they mentally transport themselves back to a healing place.

I always write in class when the students write. It is a precious, quiet time. I find my mind-mending stories always take me to Tarryall, a wide spot in the road in the Colorado Rockies, where I spent a good part of my youth, riding horses, fishing, hiking, and, well, going out to country dances on Saturday nights with the local cowboys. When my mind needs mending, I go there to our family's mountain cabin with its outdoor hand pump for water and its outhouse for other concerns.

Within a few minutes and a few words on paper, I am transported back to the high country of Colorado. I hear the ice cold and often narrow Tarryall River splash over the colorful rocks it gently smoothes as it curves through the alfalfa meadows. I see the cattails and pussy willows lining its banks.

I see my older brother, Lynn, in his plaid shirt and his rolled-up jeans.

Barehanded fishing is his specialty. He never needs a rod and reel. I see him wade barefooted into the crystal clear stream. He bends over, places his hands in the water, and waits patiently. Within minutes, a splash signals that he has caught one.

He lifts the slippery, wiggling trout from the water and tosses it onto the grassy bank. His ear-to-ear smile, verifying that he is, indeed, a mighty hunter/fisherman, brings comfort to my heart and leaves me with a sense of quiet peace. I can then re-enter the world with a mended mind.

Researchers have measured the healing power of such writing. Psychologist James W. Pennebaker, in his workbook, *Writing to Heal*, states that his research shows that expressive writing for those going through emotional upheaval can produce measurable and positive results.

"Emotional writing can also affect people's sleeping habits, work efficiency, and how they connect to others," Dr. Pennebaker writes.

In his experiments, Pennebaker's participants who wrote about traumatic experiences, were tested during and afterwards and a surprising number showed signs of reduced stress levels, better lung function in asthma patients, and even modest reductions in blood pressure. They not only felt better; they were better.

I am impressed with Dr. Pennebaker's findings.

My own observations from more than five years of teaching Writing for Wellness, although not scientific, also show that people who write about life-threatening illnesses or losing a loved one first exhibit visible signs of sadness, anger, and frustration. Some weep, choke up, and often leave the room to find a tissue. But they also return to class the next time because they say they want to continue the healing process. It seems to help.

Those who write about our topics such as healing, recapturing joy, and choosing happiness frequently smile, sigh, chuckle, and seem to relax when they finish. And, best of all, they also come back to class the next week because they say they enjoyed themselves.

Writing about mind-mending journeys has similar results. I watch it happen. As they put pen to paper, people in class look peaceful and contented. They often do not want to stop writing when time is up. They want to remain in that time and place. Following their mind-mending trips they often report feeling at peace.

The process works.

Healing Words

Bone marrow-transplant survivor Bill Matteson's class was given the mind-mending assignment. He reports taking many inner journeys while recovering.

Where Does My Mind Go to Mend?

That's an interesting question, given that the mind is a powerful tool, and it can "mend" in many ways. My mind can lead my body directly in overcoming many physical and mental ailments.

My mind actually transports me to the source of the ailment and "mends" by concentrating on the ailment and sending positive thoughts regarding its desired direction and outcome.

My mind can also help to heal indirectly by offering escape. I've been blessed with imagination and emotion, and I can visualize and experience many places and things, including how it was in times other than our own.

My mind offers relief when I let it imagine: hearing the clip-clop of horses' hooves as I ride a hansom cab down the cobblestone streets on my way to visit Sherlock Holmes at 221-B Baker Street, London; or feel a horse under me as I thunder along with my Sioux brothers on a buffalo hunt; or experience an escape to Sedona, Arizona to watch the Anasazi, the ancient ones, as they farm their fields and climb ladders to their stone houses in the cliffs; or walk to the well for a cool drink, as sentries patrol the parapets, guarding a castle.

With a creative mind, I can be anywhere and do anything. Sometimes, thinking of things in the present also offers escape. I like to mentally design a building plan, like a mantle that will frame our fireplace, or bookshelves in my office to display memories.

I also like to mentally re-order my garden so next year will be better than the present one. There is nothing more comforting, cleansing, freeing, and/or healing than a creative mind.

Think of that.

— Bill Matteson

Rick, grateful for his son's life being saved, gains solace from childhood memories.

Purity and Gratitude

Among scant memories of my early childhood, I recall once when the chill of a New England fall relented and presented a rare Indian summer day, warm enough to wander and make an "angel" in the grasses behind our yard. I looked skyward and thanked God for just being alive, warm, and secure. Alone there and aware enough at the age of perhaps four that this moment was somehow a timeout for a prayer of gratitude.

Amidst the chatter of living, I've had few pure moments of thankfulness, pauses that shed the burden of obligations and allow a rest to wash over me. But following my son's illness and long months of treatment, I wondered whether I could ever reach back again to embrace that serene moment of my childhood and rediscover what we were all meant to possess. With other souls to worry over, I now have another kind of gratitude, colored by the guilt of having been gifted my son's life, but a blessing nonetheless.

— **Rick Myers**

Robert's virtual journey transforms him.

There and Beyond

The CAT-scan confirmed my pancreatic cancer. After surgery and radiation, I was left weak and depressed. But, looking back now, I feel I died on the operating table as a caterpillar and emerged as a butterfly.

For the beauty of a butterfly is not only its appearance, but also what it has done with its life. It has traveled thousands of miles through storms and still has survived, even though it is very light and fragile.

And, it has a very short life.

I enjoy mentally visiting my family, scattered all over the garden, just like a butterfly going from flower to flower to flower.

What I have seen is similar to the beauty astronauts see when exploring space.

I have been there and beyond without ever leaving earth.

–Robert Prado.

Carole, a double stem cell-transplant survivor describes her inner journeys as she recovers.

Musings from My "Safe House"

A safe house is where:

I can enter as a child, sip on a warm cup of cocoa, and enjoy some tasty bits of freshly baked chocolate chip cookies, and be asked, "How are you really doing?" I can laugh, laugh at my mistakes or cry at my mishaps.

I can safely tell what's on my mind and forget about any cares — just like "Sesame Street." I can give myself a pat on the back and extract the best out of everything. I can sit and ponder the freshness of a word or mental image.

I can relive my favorite dream and see a barn standing boldly in polychromatic detail. What I ask of myself is only that I take a little part of this serenity and courage back into the world again.

My retreat is a tiny little room inside my safe house far away from the hustle, bustle of the world, a place free from the worries and pities of, "Why me?" a place where I can make a patchwork quilt of timeless memories, absent the gravity of expectations, rules, and demands. Where there are no demands, there are no mistakes, there are no delays, no deadlines. There is no lost time, no criticism. There are no missed chances. Here in my safety zone, I'm free.

— Carole Palmquist

Annie's refuge renews her and reminds her of what is important.

A Place I Go

There's a place that I go when I'm feeling down,
　and the cares of the world get the best of me.
When I'm wondering why I'm here,
　and I feel I've misplaced the rest of me.
When my day's been the pits, I long to crawl into bed
　and stay with the covers pulled over my head,
　there's a place that I go.
It's in the healing echoes of my children's laughter
　that my heart finds rest that my soul longs after.
It's in the wisdom of their gentle teasing
　or their reassurance that I find so pleasing.
Since first gazing into their new-born eyes
　I've been their champion and they've been mine.
If I had not been blessed to have them as children,
　I would surely want them as my very best friends.

— Annie Watson

It's Your Turn

Although it may be impossible to travel far away while recovering from major illness or tragedy, it is not impossible to send your mind away for repairs. Instead of watching endless violence and conflict on the television, take a paper and pen to a quiet place. Close your eyes and let your mind find the most peaceful moment it can locate. When you are there, open your eyes and begin to describe what you see, hear, taste, smell, and feel. Your body may become relaxed and your pain may not be as severe for a while as you see vivid colors of landscapes you have experienced or feel the salt spray on your face from a crashing wave on the beach. Write about why you think your mind chose that particular memory.

Jump Start

I will never forget the feeling I had when I (saw, visited, experienced) ...

I choose to leave sadness, pain, and sorrow behind as I return to the day when ...

Following your writing, how did you feel? Did it help relax you and take some of your stress away? If so, you may want to consciously take a mind-mending journey from time to time. It has to be less stressful than watching the news.

Chapter 18

Recapturing Joy

I danced on the moon one night and the stars twinkled with me.

— Robyn Bryson

When tragedy or major illnesses strike, your life is turned upside down. Doctors, surgeries, and family members take away your privacy, and the lack of schedules and routines combine to create chaos and upheaval. Add pain and uncertainty and it is no wonder your life is stressful.

With sadness sometimes consuming you, it doesn't seem possible to see beyond your tears and fears. The weight of your situation may almost immobilize you.

You may long to feel moments of happiness, but in your present circumstances, you may feel that is almost impossible.

It isn't.

It can take a concerted effort to get joy back into your mind. But, to recapture those positive, joyful times, it is necessary to consciously push

200

the sadness away from your way of thinking, at least for short periods.

When you want to escape to happier times through writing, you can accomplish this by following some simple steps:

1. Force yourself to go back mentally to a time in your life when you felt pure joy. It may have been watching the birth of your child, standing on the stage at your graduation, having your grandfather read to you, seeing the sunrise over the Grand Canyon, reuniting with a lost love, or fulfilling your life dream of seeing one of your heroes in a live concert or a sports event. You may want to recall a camping trip, a school play, a great vacation, a favorite pet, or special holiday with family.

2. Choose one particular experience. Close your eyes for a minute or two and transport yourself back. How does that moment feel? Can you recall what people are saying? How did you look, feel? Can you describe the sounds, the sights? Are you able to capture any or all of the feelings you have at that place or time? Take time to write down any and all details and feelings you recall. Write in the present tense, "I see..." "I feel..." "I hear..."

If you can recapture those moments in your imagination, you can write about them and, in doing so, relive them. After this exercise, try to remember that you can recapture the joy you have experienced even when you are in the most unlikely places and under some highly usual circumstances.

3. When undergoing chemotherapy or having a scan of some kind, instead of being afraid or sad, take that time to concentrate on and then relive a joyful moment. If you have to remain perfectly still, as when having some medical procedures or treatment, you may discover that it is the perfect time to recapture special moments.

In class, when I tell students to return to a place where they feel joy and a time when happiness and pleasure are abundant, I watch them as they write. Their faces slowly change from stoic or grim to peaceful and happy. It works. Just like chicken soup. It works every time. It will work for you. Some people write about special memories when loved ones who have passed away were with them. Despite some initial sadness, they write about the happy days and cherished moments. A night to remember, a first love, an engagement party — all special memories that people choose. If the memory is private, there is no need to share the writing with anyone.

Healing Words

Bill selects memories of childhood to transform him from a bone marrow transplant patient back to being a carefree kid.

Ghosts of Halloweens Past

Halloween was a lot of fun when I was growing up. I guess it is for children today, too, but in the 1950s, Halloween was also safe. We didn't have to watch out for things that could harm us possibly being put into our candy, and we often received fruit or cookies for our treats, things that today's kids would probably scoff at.

We could trick or treat wherever we could manage to walk to, and our parents never went along to chaperone. It was a wonderful time.

It was magical.

When I was seven, my father changed jobs, and we moved to a trailer park in a small town in western New York. I enjoyed it a lot, especially on Halloween; there were a lot of families in a relatively small area. We'd go trick-or-treating for a couple of hours and, in that time, I'd usually fill two or three grocery bags with candy, fruit, cookies, and popcorn balls.

Things changed a little when I became a teenager. At this point, on Halloween, all the kids would meet downtown at the main shopping area where hundreds of other teenagers gathered, most of them armed with water balloons or shaving cream, or both. We'd come home wet, cold, and sticky. Still, those memories are a joy.

One year I'll never forget was when it was raining cats and dogs, and we were all out in it anyway.

Someone had made a straw dummy that looked suspiciously like the football coach at our rival high school, and had hung it from a downtown overpass. Where the overpass crossed it, the street itself dipped down about six feet and there was a drain on one side at the bottom to prevent flooding.

One of the rival school's students took offense at their "coach" dangling off the viaduct, and in his wisdom, cut him down, causing the dummy to fall and plug up the drain. The street soon filled with water up to the level of the sidewalk. Of course, hometown drivers, seeing this and knowing how deep the water was, stopped and took a detour.

But, sad to say, the driver of a little red Volkswagen with Canadian plates ventured on. It wasn't more than a heartbeat before the VW was floating. It then proceeded to the middle of the water, turned sideways, and stopped. Unsure of what to do, the perplexed driver opened the door to get out, and the car immediately sank, with only a few inches of its roof left showing.

My last memory is of the driver bailing out the inside of his car with a hubcap.

— Bill Matteson

Caregivers of the terminally ill, like Gordon, often need to care for themselves in order to bring joy and balance back into their lives.

Childhood Treasures

My mind possesses the power to make life's unpleasant realities become far more endurable. While waiting in a doctor's office, I use that power to mentally transport myself back in time. I go back to a better time and a better place, to days with my father, my mother, my older brother, days at the seashore. I hear the waves, smell the sea salt. I can see my parents, my brother. I can hear their voices. Suddenly, I feel at peace; I feel joy. Even today, the sights and sounds of those wonderful symbols — beach balls, toy sailboats with their bleached-white, stretched-out sails rising high above the miniaturized decks, or even the sight of gaudy beach towels help take me away from life's stresses.

Will I ever again feel so carefree, so in love with life?

— Gordon Dyer

Annie served as a caregiver for her terminally ill boyfriend. Still, when asked to write about recapturing joy, she was able to relive love-filled moments.

Remembering You

Each time I call to mind the love we shared,
Those precious times, reality is soon retreated.
Thoughts of you grow sweeter still.
My heart will hold them fresh until
I see your face and feel completed.
My face cupped in your hands,
I smile a breathless kiss.
You hold me while my love is overflowing.
Finger kisses wave goodbye.

I taste your tears each time you cry.
Within your arms, my fears are going.
Bring me back to days gone by.
When warm winds come, I hear your sigh.
Perfect love my heart is holding.
Now saints and angels will know your charms,
As you wake up in your Father's arms,
You final wish now unfolding.

— Annie Watson

Edna, who sings in professional choral groups in the Los Angeles area, vividly recalls hearing one special word from her childhood that was truly music to her ears.

Choose Me

I vividly remember a moment of pure joy that happened when I was in the third grade. It was long ago, yet I still get goose bumps when I think about it.

We are in class, sitting at our long communal tables that serve as desks. A visitor enters our classroom. I recognize her as Miss Abel, our elementary school's music teacher.

My teacher, Miss Plough, interrupts her lesson and, clapping her hands and briskly announcing, "Attention, children! Miss Abel is here to select students to sing in our school chorus.

"She will give you a song to sing. If she pats you on the shoulder as she walks by, that means you have been chosen.

"If that happens, come to the front of the class and stand quietly."

I can't believe my ears. Here is my chance to sing in the school chorus! I will actually make music with the other children, with Miss Abel leading us.

The thought fills me with such excitement I can hardly sit still.

Silently, I start to pray — "Please, let her choose me! Please, please, please, I want to sing! Please, please, please!"

As we begin our audition song, I watch Miss Abel's every movement with intense interest. She slowly walks up and down the aisles, critically listening to each voice.

When she touches a child's shoulder, it is as though she has turned Cinderella from the servant girl into the princess.

She starts to come down my aisle.

"Please, oh please!" I plead with whomever or whatever had the power to intercede with Miss Abel on my behalf.

After what seems an eternity, she passes me and I feel the slightest tap on my shoulder. I am stunned.

Have I imagined it, or is it real? I look up at Miss Abel.

She smiles at me and whispers, "Yes."

I want to run and scream with a sense of delicious, intense joy. I have been chosen. I am special.

As an adult, I have sung in prominent choral groups and always counted my blessings for being able to participate. But nothing comes close to recapturing the joy of that moment, so long ago, when Miss Abel gave me my voice.

— Edna Teller

Shannon, whose childhood tragedies could have consumed her, consciously chose the joy of imagined places and fantasy to carry her away from reality and help her heal.

Glitterbows

Hollow voices speak to me,
In illusions of my sleep,
To tell me things of no importance,
And wish me not to weep.
Of adventures on a magic horse,
Cantering in the sky.
And miracles of caterpillars,
That explode to butterflies.
For inner peace to choose my world,
And keep it close at heart,
To understand my realm is there,
And we'll never be apart.
Wishes putting names with faces,
Of figures that lift me high,
From my bed to a fantasy stream,
Of strudel-colored skies.
So I'll name them "glitterbows,"
As it's the farthest I can go,
To remember with my eyes aloft
Of stained rainbows on my soul.

— Shannon Lynn Marshall

Joan writes about newfound joy that came when she least expected it.

Millennium Magic

The year 2000, hailed joyfully by many, had a most inauspicious beginning for me. January brought my mastectomy, followed by months of chemotherapy, culminating in nine weeks of radiation through the end of October.

Simultaneously, the loving, caring, and supportive man in my life began the slow, cruel slide toward the fearful, cold, and self-absorbed individual that Alzheimer's would ultimately create. Nowhere in that scenario could I envision joy.

The months ahead held only uncertainty. Then, when an invitation to a family wedding arrived, I considered it carefully. Perhaps this would be my final opportunity to participate in such a positive family gathering, and to see the sisters, nieces, nephews, and cousins that I loved.

I accepted the invitation on behalf of myself and my 18-year-old granddaughter who had never been to the East Coast, nor met many of the members of her extended family. Without being aware of it, I had made a wise move.

The plane ride provided a rare opportunity to visit with Emily one-on-one. Emily and her family live outside Los Angeles in the mountains; I live in the flatlands. Our trip marked the beginning of a closeness between us that had not existed previously.

It was a wonderful week, and I began to feel the beginning of a hopefulness that there would be more to come.

When I got home, my then six-year-old grandson sat beside me at dinner.

"We missed you, Grandma," he told me. "Everybody loves you."

The glow I felt then was enhanced by his next remark. "Take off your hat, Grandma. I love to see your bald head."

Oh, joy! Welcome back to my life.

— **Joan Smith**

It's Your Turn

Let your mind help you escape the negatives. Then, when you get a few free moments, write about the happiness you once felt. Keep a small notebook and pen handy. Very few people will interrupt you when you are busily writing, whether it is in a waiting room, your hospital room, or your living room. If someone starts to divert your attention, merely hold up your hand and signal for them to allow you to complete your thoughts. Closing your eyes helps you to get privacy, too. If you liked school, think of a favorite teacher. Try to picture him or her. Was there a special moment you recall?

Write in detail about the joy you felt. Describe what took place, paying close attention to your five senses. What was the weather like? What sensations did you feel physically? We all acknowledge that unhappy memories can bring tears to our eyes and we know that scary movies or thrill rides at the carnival can frighten us, making our hearts race and our hands tremble. Doesn't it make sense that remembering happy moments can bring joy to our hearts?

Jump Start

I feel joy, pure joy when I remember ...

One of the best memories in my life was when ...

See if you can find peace by mentally returning to a place that made you feel wonderful. Take a deep breath, and remember a time in your life when everything was calm. Think about it as being here and now.

Then write in the present tense about what you see, feel, hear.

I can feel the peace and quiet surround me as I remember ....

After you have finished writing, share that writing with someone close to you by reading it aloud to him or her.

This might be someone who may not know about this experience or someone who actually was there at the time. Either way, the listener will see your joy emerge and you may feel your stress evaporate.

Chapter 19

Smiling through the Tears

*Even during tragedy, things happen to provide
us with comic relief.*

— Jeff Howe

My mother's hospital room in Boulder, Colorado, holds many
memories for me. Some are tragic; others make me laugh out loud.

On her first day in the hospital, the doctor walked in, a man who was
a Doogie Howser look-alike, only younger. This guy looked 12.

My mother, then in her 70s, was from the old school. She was born
in the South. She always wore a hat and gloves when she traveled on a
train and always dressed up for airplane trips. She wouldn't go to the
store in slacks or shorts, and she always wore an apron when she was
preparing dinner. Her earrings were ever-present, a little like Barbara
Bush and her pearls.

With those she knew she couldn't have been more fun or more
relaxed. She loved people. But she could be rather formal when speaking
to doctors, bankers, or other professionals she was meeting for the first

time.

Even as a small child, I noticed her language and demeanor immediately changed when our insurance man came to the door or someone from the county government, such as the tax assessor, rang our doorbell.

She expected to be treated rather formally by strangers, too. It was just the way it was. After all, she was born in 1909.

So, when a stranger, a young doctor, with his ever-so-modern ways entered her hospital room and extended his hand saying, "Hello, there, how are we?" adding, "I'm your doctor," I knew it wasn't going to go over well.

His tone was rather patronizing, something my mother could pick up a mile away.

As he came closer, she pulled the covers up to her chin. Clearly, this boy was not going to put his hands on her.

He stopped and checked his clipboard, noticing her unusual first name.

"And you are, let me see, it is Mozelle? May I call you Mozelle?"

My mother, suffering the first stages of senility took one look at him, stiffened, and said in a slightly arrogant tone as if speaking to one of the neighborhood kids, "No. No you may not. You may call me Mrs. Bolger."

The doctor was flustered and kind of sputtered after that, taking his stethoscope from around his neck and leaning over her. He performed a cursory exam, trying to check her pulse and listen to her heart. All the while my mother lay staring at him with suspicion. It was obvious that she didn't think he was a real doctor and wondered why he was fiddling around with her. The outrage of it all.

I could barely keep from laughing at the two of them.

My brother, sister-in-law, and I were all on edge. Just the day before, my niece had been helping my mother bathe in her assisted-living apartment when Teri, who later became a nurse, discovered a large lump on my mother's breast.

An exam revealed that both breasts were involved and she was put into the hospital immediately. Her doctor feared the tumors were cancerous.

Ironically, once she was admitted to the hospital, my mother didn't realize that she was even a patient. She thought I was and kept telling me how she hoped I'd get well soon.

As conflicted as we were, her comments made us smile, even through our tears.

I stayed all night with her the first night, sleeping in a large chair in her room. I feared that she might awaken and panic, not knowing where or even who she was. She woke up a couple of times, saw me, and again tried to comfort me.

"Gee, honey, I hope they find out what's wrong with you!"

In the middle of the night, a nurse came in. I must admit, the woman was most unattractive, very large, and she had a booming raspy voice. (Maybe that's why she was on the night shift.) I woke with a start as soon as I heard her speak.

She leaned over my mother's bed and said rather harshly, "I'm here to check your vitals," her face coming very close to my mother's.

Mom sat up and screamed, "Get away from me! You are SO ugly! So ugly!" I jumped from my chair and tried to intercede. It was too late. The nurse looked angrily at me.

I explained, "She's not herself! I'm so sorry!"

The nurse sighed and quickly left the room. Mom laid back down, looked as if she had merely experienced a bad dream, and rolled over.

Early the next morning, another nurse came in with a small plastic container with a lid on it. It had my mother's name printed on it along with a barcode.

The nurse came to my mother's bed side and said, "Mrs. Bolger? We'll need a sample," gesturing to the adjoining bathroom as she placed the container on the tray table. My mother frowned at it, picked it up, and looked at the barcode, squinting as if she had never seen one before.

"Sample?" she asked, looking at the nurse and then at me for help.

"You know, Mom, a urine sample? You have to go in that container."

My mother looked totally disgusted, placed the container on her tray table, and kind of pushed it away from her.

"Why in heaven's name would I want to go in that little thing when there is a perfectly good toilet right over there?"

The nurse and I locked eyes and smiled.

Mom had a good point.

Healing Words

Hospitals, doctors, illnesses — nothing very funny about them on the surface. But talk to a few patients or their families and you can't help smiling. Those unforgettable and even embarrassing moments can bring the laughter back — weeks, months, and even years later. Sometimes even a belly laugh spills out when a particular memory surfaces.

Laughter often provides a release from tension. You can laugh so hard you cry. Or you can cry so hard you laugh.

Lois was getting her doctorate. Her husband was dying of cancer and her mother no longer recognized her. What's funny about that?

Keep Smiling

My advice on how to survive what life throws at you is to keep going despite the bumps, curves, ditches, detours, and unpaved roads and focus your attention and love outward and keep smiling!

Four surgeries, internal radiation, four rounds of chemotherapy, hair lost three times, loss of a husband and father, a Mom diagnosed with dementia, and loss of close friends from cancer aren't the easiest of challenges while I've battled ovarian cancer. But I have survived for 15 years and have traveled a road with many curves, detours, and bumps, but also have had 15 years of experiencing some of the journey's finest moments. However, no matter what one does, accepts, rejects, or stalls, one has to realize life still travels at high speed and time is running out. If the journey is to be filled with as much love, positive happenings, feelings of warmth and appreciation as possible, the navigator (you/me to be exact) has to focus externally on God, friends, family, and the world and refuse to get stuck in the muck of self-pity and remorse.

I'd like to tell you a story. It's bittersweet, poignant, sad, hilarious, emotional — all at the same time. It's May 29th, graduation day and I am getting my doctorate. Mickey and Walter, my Mom and Dad, flew to California from New Jersey to witness my graduation. However, it wasn't all joyous, light, and happy as my husband Bill was at the City of Hope struggling with throat cancer, radiation, rounds of chemotherapy, and no platelet count.

Friends had already donated platelets, but it was still touch and go. Because of this turn of events, my planned, big graduation celebration was canceled. Fortunately, as the weekend approached, a few close friends and two cousins rushed in to help Bill and me. After some discussion about celebrating this occasion, we decided to bring the party to Bill at the City of Hope after the graduation ceremony.

The day started out like a circus — crazy and zany. My cousin's wife, Kathie, said she would take care of Mickey (who was in early stages of dementia) and help her get dressed and steer her through the day. Walter, my Dad, was trying to be as helpful as a host to the visiting relatives and guests who were staying at the house. I was nervous and excited as I had to make a speech that day, but also happy I had some hair and didn't have to wear my wig.

At 11 a.m. we attended pre-ceremony activities. All went fine until we reached the La Verne University campus, and I realized that I had lost my gold watch, which had been given to me by Bill when I had defended my dissertation.

I was distraught. Mom didn't know what was happening. Dad didn't know what to do, but cousins Carol and Bob volunteer to return to the Pomona Complex and see if they could find my watch.

As the music began and I marched into the arena in cap and gown, tears were flowing. Dad and Kathie were holding on to my Mom, and the ceremony was proceeding. Halfway through the speeches to which I was scarcely paying attention, Carol with this huge smile on her face sneaked down the aisle, attracted my eye, and waved the watch in the air.

Someone had found it and turned it in to the hotel desk. She picked it up and dashed back to the graduation, as she knew I would feel happy and relieved if I saw it. To this day, I don't know the angel who found my watch. I can never say thank you enough to that very honest person.

What feelings of gratitude, love, and affection I had for this stranger and, naturally, for my cousin Carol.

But the most touching scene came the day following graduation. We all packed into our cars and drove to the City of Hope to see Bill and drink a toast for the occasion. Even though he couldn't attend the graduation, all of us wanted him to be part of the day's celebration. Seven of us crowded into his room with gowns and masks and sneaked in two bottles of chilled champagne with glasses for everyone.

Since we were a noisy crowd as we cheered and sipped champagne, we attracted inquisitive visitors. Sure enough, as he was completing his daily rounds, Bill's doctor and his team appeared and asked, "Oh, What's this? Do we smell alcohol?"

It certainly was a pregnant moment as we thought we were in deep trouble. But, when the doctor heard the explanation of our celebration, he laughed and said, "Have a good time and enjoy."

And this is the way we went about our lives, living with cancer. We did the best we could under some very challenging circumstances. But, we tried to laugh, celebrate, love, give our thanks to God, family and friends for helping us navigate life's highway.

— Dr. Lois W. Neil

Dave was exhausted, ready to give up. Against his doctor's judgment, he had taken himself off chemotherapy and decided not to continue to fight his cancer, but then something happened.

Being Barney

Taking myself off chemotherapy the week before turned out to be a positive psychological step for me. I felt that, for the first time going through this whole cancer ordeal, I was in control.

But I decided to return a week later and was in a better state of mind to accept chemo treatments again. In fact, I started singing, very loudly and probably off key a little to poke fun at my situation.

I'm not sure everyone within the sound of my voice appreciated it.

(Sung to Barney's theme song tune)

"I love chemo, Chemo loves me,

We're just one big fam-a-lee..."

My next chest scans showed that the tumors in my lungs had shrunk by 37%, and the subsequent scan of my head showed that the cancer tumors in my brain were all gone. In fact, the doctors said my head was empty.

Of course we all knew that.

— David Key

In England, even on her deathbed with her grieving relatives surrounding her, Elizabeth's mother had the last laugh.

Recollections of Mother

My mother passed away on Mother's Day in the year 2000. As a child growing up, I couldn't see many similarities between us. She had dark wavy hair, brown eyes, and the fairest of complexions. I was blonde with green eyes and I tanned easily. In fact, one day a woman came up to my mother when my brother and I were small and commended my mother for not only adopting one child but the sibling, too!

My mother was small while I was tall. In school my mother was a high achiever academically and captain of her cricket team. I did well academically but excelled in all sports.

My mother was a voracious reader who loved to talk about books so much she started her own book club in 1975. I liked to read, but could never understand how she could enjoy reading and re-reading the same book over time especially when the title of the book was *Death Be Not Proud*. She compared it to seeing the same play twice "You always discover something new the second time around," she would say.

She was a great raconteur and the life of the party, loved going to the theater and taking drives in the countryside. She also insisted on good manners and properly spoken English "It's 'do you have,' not 'have you got!' You can't be very unique; you're either unique or you're not."

She was a strict disciplinarian. When she discovered my brother as a teenager was growing marijuana in her upstairs study, she threatened to call the police. And when he didn't comply with her demand that it should be removed, she did call the police. He had just enough time to switch the marijuana plants for other plants that he was cultivating and never tried that venture again.

She always spoke her mind no matter what the circumstances. One friend described her as ruthlessly honest.

While she was at home nearing death, resting on the bed where she would die, she suddenly spoke out very loudly, "I'm dying, I'm dying, I'm dying!" Not expecting such an outburst, my siblings and stepfather all looked at one another in horror. We all leaned forward and gasped.

"I'm dying for a cigarette!" she exclaimed with a hoot of laugher that we shall never forget, especially since she never smoked a cigarette in her life.

— Elizabeth Terry

The writing class had been assigned to write about the topic "It was the best of times; it was the worst of times" during their cancer experiences. What had they endured? How had they changed because of it? I gave them some quiet time to think and then to begin writing. Most participants looked serious and wrote poignant pieces about how they had coped or how they fell apart at certain times. Not Joy. She had a grin on her face the entire time as her Braille machine clicked and clacked rapidly. Clearly, she knew what she wanted to say. Nobody was ready for what she wrote.

If anyone could find something funny about breast cancer surgery, it would be Joy. She had often shared with the group that her mastectomy had left her longing to be "normal" again. We were not surprised when she came to class months earlier and had been to a surgeon. Joy had a solution. A "tram-flap" operation would take her skin, fat, and tissue from her tummy area and move it up to create a new breast, she hoped, making her whole again. She couldn't wait to have it done. There would be no foreign material to be rejected. There would be no breast implants to collapse down the line. Joy had the operation and was thrilled with her results.

But that day, after the Dickens' quotation was read and the class had finished writing, Joy's hand went up and she immediately stood to recite, barely able contain her laughter. The title alone caused pandemonium in the classroom.

The Tale of Two Titties

It was the best of times. It was the worst of times.

Teetee and Boobie were twins, though not identical. Teetee was bigger and remained so throughout their natural life. These girls were very close as they grew up. They shared the carefree days of early childhood. They remained close during their teenage years when, together, they endured the embarrassment of crude men's digs. Their companionship lasted even through childbearing and nursing.

One day, a terrible thing happened. Boobie was taken away, never to be seen again. How Teetee mourned her loss! Though she had a family, she could not endure the loss of her twin. So she headed south in search of a companion.

After several years had elapsed, Teetee heard that a companion had been found. She allowed herself to be brought back from down South. Imagine her joy when she met her new companion. She looked almost like Boobie. She felt warm and alive. Teetee was thrilled. She had been so lonely. It wasn't Boobie, but it was as close as she would ever get to having a bosom buddy again.

Teetee's contentment with her new companion is often ruffled by the thought that what happened to Boobie could someday happen to her, too. However, when these thoughts invade her mind, she thrusts them aside, trusting in God that it will not be so.

For now, she will enjoy her new companion and revel in the gifts that each new day brings.

— Joy E. Walker Steward

Jodie's mother was in grave condition. The family had gathered at her hospital bedside. No one expected her to regain consciousness or live through the day. But, when her doctor entered her room, those around her were surprised by her words.

Heavenly Destination?

When Dr. Vannis, mother's physician, came into her room, Mother was completely still. We didn't expect her to notice or even move, but she suddenly opened her eyes widely and stated very clearly, "Well, hello, Doctor Vannis! I didn't know you were on this airplane."

— Jodie Davis

(Alma Hall, 84, died later that day.)

Sally King, in her mid 60s, and retired Los Angeles Fire Department Assistant Chief Bill Durkee were part of a group of about 60 senior citizens who met at the YMCA each weekday morning at 8 a.m. for water aerobics classes. Sally and Bill both enjoyed a good joke. She loved listening to them; he loved telling them. While the other participants were splashing through the exercises, Bill would slip up behind Sally while she was talking with friends and quietly say "Boo!" Sally would jump every time, turn around, and get ready for the day's laugh.

After a few years of attending classes, Sally showed up at the pool with large bruises on her arms. She told Bill the bad news. She had developed an acute and virulent leukemia. Bill and others at the pool kept contact while she ran the gamut of chemo, radiation, and finally bone marrow transplant after total body radiation. She fought the good fight, but finally had to tell her pool buddies that the doctors had taken back her "get out of jail" card, and there was no longer any hope. Sally told them she was checking into a hospice and didn't expect to be there long. Bill wanted to say goodbye, to tell her his feelings, and used humor in the following note.

A Friend's Farewell

Well, Sally, it looks like you're going to see heaven before I am. Now when you approach the Pearly Gates, you tell Saint Peter that Bill Durkee said to put you in there with the angels, because they can use a little humor up there!

While you're at it, look around the fences there and see if there's a crack somewhere. I know when I get there, my only chance is if you help pull me through a crack. I think the only reason they leave me down here is to serve as a bad example.

Well, it's been a good ride.

Love ya, "Boo Billy"

— Bill Durkee

Chuck Bergman was trying to make lemonade out of the lemons his family had been given when his wife Linda, a successful Hollywood writer/producer, was diagnosed with leukemia. She could die. She was undergoing treatment that was supposed to stop her cancer, but instead had created somewhat of a new personality.

Sometimes Chuck was torn between laughing and crying.

Hitting the Bull's-Eye at Target

Now a regular in cancer treatment, Linda refused to be put "under" for marrow aspirations because she would not give up a couple of days of her writing. Ativan was fine, she told her doctors.

"Just a couple of hours in twilight, a night's sleep and I'll be back at it," she explained.

Except for that Target store near City of Hope. They have everything you do and don't need, want and don't want.

"It's soooo inviting!" she'd tell me.

I tried to protest. She never stopped at Target. She needed to get well. But she insisted that she must immediately be taken to Target. There was no arguing. I acquiesced.

I drove her to Target and she enthusiastically raced through the store with the gusto of a kid in a candy store, eyes scanning each item, her mouth almost watering with delight.

A pair of loose pants for summer would be good! Maybe a top also.

Great! You can just toss them on in the aisles. No need for fitting rooms or privacy.

Most shoppers also take one item off before trying on the next, and the next, and the next.

Most people in Target aren't on Ativan.

Picture a small child bundled up for a winter outing, arms held upright by layers of shirts, sweaters, and coats. Legs plumped by thermals. A five-foot, four-inch child.

Linda "needed" them all, and, as we peeled them off her at the checkout register, the cashier looked on in wonder.

$135 buys a lot of summer garments at Target.

The next morning, the inevitable.

"Where did all these clothes come from?"

— Chuck Bergman

Violet's sense of humor never ceased to amaze those around her. Even when hospitalized in France after a tragic automobile accident, she found time to laugh at her own American hang-ups and how they conflicted with those of La Francaise.

La Bassine Francaise

When confined to any hospital, the only 100% way to guarantee the arrival of your doctor or a visitor, regardless of the time — night or day — is for you to be on the bedpan.

So open to public scrutiny, I always felt insecure while sitting on "la bassine" as it is called, while I was confined to a hospital in France.

Direct contact with an aluminum, porcelain, or enamel pan at one end while trying to emit gracious repartee from the other just did not relax me.

I always delayed as long as possible the unavoidable call of nature.

One day my daughter Elaine, who was also badly injured in the accident and was sharing the hospital room with me, was waiting to be taken off "le trone" (the throne) as the younger nurses called it, when we heard our doctor's voice down the hall.

We knew he was bringing other doctors with him for a consultation on Elaine's condition before her scheduled surgery.

Against all hospital rules, I managed to roll quickly out of my bed, grab her full bedpan, and slip it under the foot of Elaine's bed.

I got back under my covers just as the door opened and three dignified doctors walked into our room.

Such perfect timing had left us both a little breathless. It was also the first time since the accident that Elaine had felt light-hearted enough for a little laugh.

While the physicians encircled my daughter's bed, making a thorough examination of her fractures, charts, and traction equipment, the head nun stood by holding x-rays and instruments. It was a serious and dignified occasion with French medical terms and diagnoses batted back and forth across Elaine's bed like a dizzy ball in the heat of a table-tennis championship.

As the doctors picked up their medical-bag miscellany in preparation to leave, Dr. Musselon stepped closer to Elaine to take one last look.

He put his foot under the bed and it came out encircled by the bedpan.

What a noise he made when he shouted and shook his foot, liquid wildly splashing everywhere before the pan left his shoe and clanked to the floor making a puddle!

What a picture he made poised on one foot furiously shaking the other!

The nun ran from the room returning with towels and a mop.

I looked at Elaine in horror and then we both laughed — evidently the wrong thing to do. The other French doctors took one disgusted look at the two of us, held their heads high, and marched out of our room.

I can assure you that French-American relations have never before nor since been more strained than at that moment.

But after three days of not seeing the offended doctor, we inquired and learned that we needed to formally apologize for laughing at him because the doctor's professional pride had been injured and he would not return to treat us.

We were informed by a young intern that we needed to explain that we were laughing at the entire incident, not at the doctor himself. We contacted the doctor, made our apologies, and quickly got back in his good graces.

We did get a lecture though. An American doctor informed us about la bassine, which is never hidden in France but is as boldly displayed as a glass of water. Had we not visited the public restrooms in Paris, shared without a moment's hesitancy by both men and women?

We learned that our puritanical American ideas were pedantic and unknown in France. I wondered how I had grown to womanhood with so much false modesty.

Once again on good terms with our doctor, from then on either Elaine or I was always comfortably getting on or off a basin during his visits.

We also learned graciously and gracefully to condition ourselves to remain seated on our basins and to hide our secret predicaments from visitors who gathered at the tea hour to share their French pastries and homemade teacakes with us. The hospital aides, meanwhile, were too busy serving tea and coffee to patients and guests to be summoned for such ordinary chores as basin removal.

La bassine was only one link in the uninhibited French life. Shined like diamonds, always warmed before being presented to patients, covered with embroidered cloths to keep them warm, they were always offered by beautiful young smiling nurses who pleaded affectionately, "Take one please."

I can at last shout with sincere approval, "Viva La France! Viva La Bassine!"

— Violet Wightman

It's Your Turn

After having read the stories above, do you remember anything funny happening during your interactions with those in the medical world? If so, describe in as much detail as you can a humorous incident you witnessed in a doctor's office or hospital or at home during a relative's illness. Perhaps it involved a child who didn't understand the procedure. Provide as many descriptions and direct quotes as you can recall. This will make the readers feel as though they were there, too.

Jump Start

The funniest thing that ever happened while in the hospital/doctor's office was ...

I'll never forget the look on ...'s face when ...

Remembering the humorous times may not speed up your recovery but it may make things a bit less depressing.

Chapter 20

Capturing Nature's Power

I see dancing daffodils
among mountain wildflowers.
I see mighty eagles soaring
through wispy clouds

— Carole Palmquist

As far back as I can remember, my parents took me to the mountains — to fish, to ride in a boat, to have a picnic, to visit eccentrics my father knew, to cool off from the summer's heat, to see the aspens turning, to watch the first snow fall, to sled and toboggan and ski, and always to see the first wildflowers of spring.

Living in Colorado Springs, at the foot the 14,000-foot giant, Pikes Peak, the nearby mountains were our weather gauge, our entertainment, our air conditioner, and our signal of the seasons. Dark clouds and lightning over "the Peak" meant rain; swirling white clouds and fog around its summit meant snow; and splashes of golden aspens whipping in warm Chinook winds on its face meant summer was over.

Before my parents had much money to spare, they drove to the mountains with a picnic dinner and a fishing pole several times a week in the summer or early fall. After my father got off work at the wholesale floral company, he would pick up my mother at the telephone company office downtown where she was a long-distance operator, and with my brother and me in the backseat, we'd head up Ute Pass.

Mom loved not having to cook every night and my father preferred fishing to eating anyway. My older brother and I went along for the ride at first and then both grew to love the outdoors.

Sometimes, in fact oftentimes, we would have to eat meals inside our car due to rain or hail or snow. Colorado, to those who know her, is capricious, always keeping her residents guessing. But the message my parents taught us, without ever verbalizing it, was that to commune with nature was healing. The stress of the day could be erased by watching a magpie strut around a picnic site, by pulling a rainbow trout out of a rushing stream, by seeing a big-horned sheep cling to a rocky mountainside, or by just rolling down the car windows to hear the meadowlarks tuning up. We always came back home feeling better than when we left. Nature's healing power was magical.

After my father started his own flower business and put away some cash, he and my mother bought a small mountain cabin in Tarryall, about an hour and a half's drive from Colorado Springs, the last 10 miles of which were on a bumpy dirt road that paralleled the Tarryall River.

The cabin was not a resort. It had one large room, a wood stove, a Murphy bed that came down from the wall, and a "loft" that was accessed by a built-in wooden ladder attached to one wall. There was no kitchen sink, no bathroom, and not much insulation. It was cold in the winter, hot in the summer. But, to us, it was a palace, outhouse and all.

For the 20 years that we went to the cabin — first the original one and then a somewhat nicer, larger one just up the hill — we had countless memorable times together. Soon after my parents bought the second cabin, all of our relatives came, too. It was not unusual to have a dozen or so of our immediate family — all four grandparents, first cousins, aunts, and uncles. There was still no running water or inside toilet.

Everyone wanted to go to the cabin for the same reason — to get away. And every time, the mountains worked their magic. A hike, a stroll along a stream, a meal outside under a pine tree, a glimpse of a deer, a bobcat, or a beaver building his winter home took us from the stress of the week into the glory of nature.

My husband and I are avid hikers. We have visited most of the national parks in this country and some in Canada and Europe. Friends ask us what we do when we get there. We tell them we look and hike. Then we hike and look. When our vacation is over, we feel better — lots better.

So, when my students in Writing for Wellness come in stressed and sad, I prescribe a visit with Mother Nature. Sometimes, because of disabilities, they are unable to physically go anywhere. Travel videos allow them to see places they haven't seen and revisit some they have. They are also a good jumping off place to begin writing.

On the City of Hope's more than 1,200-acre grounds there are numerous places to sit to enjoy nature. Benches are positioned on lawns, in rose gardens, and near waterfalls to allow families and patients to contemplate and heal. There is also a Japanese garden with flowers, a waterfall, and streams emptying into a koi pond. Rabbits, birds, squirrels and even an occasional coyote can be seen on the grounds.

When I ask students to write about how nature has helped heal them, many in the class enthusiastically begin to write even before we have our pre-writing time when ideas are exchanged. Once they hear the topic, they have their ideas and they are off and writing.

Healing Words

Rick, an avid swimmer, who, no matter the weather, does laps five days a week at the outside pool near the Rose Bowl, jumped right in to write about how the sea welcomes and refreshes him during his summer visits to Martha's Vineyard Island.

Swimmingly Simple

My adult "time-out," far from being punitive, satisfies a primal need to become grounded. Retreating to golf is perhaps a more popular bromide, but it requires financial commitment, equipment, and considerable self-management, all in all a rather elaborate method for restoration. More simple is a swim in the sea.

Ocean swimming precludes cell phones, club dues, and competition. A saline solution is the most compatible environment for the human constitution, and presents a basic return to our origins.

For me it both heals and energizes. Some swims begin in discomfort, the initial chill jolting me out of whatever thoughts I came with — the muted world of the sea, allowing no sounds other than the hum of my exertion; tasting salt; breathing rhythmically to avoid oxygen debt; surging occasionally or varying my dance to create an imagined threat or to push a new pulse of exhilaration.

The sun comforts, but only the top layer, and illuminates the sands and seaweed below, offering the illusion of flight over a world devoid of human corruption, colored by nature, choreographed by her graceful suspension of creatures without air.

I can draw myself anew in these visits to a silent world.

— Rick Myers

The class was worried about Robert. We could see he was losing weight; his skin looked pale. He didn't have the bounce in his step that was his trademark. When he told us he was going in for CAT scans and blood tests, he looked concerned. We all hoped his cancer hadn't come back.

A Miracle with Help

For three months I had not felt very well. In those three months, I had symptoms of the 24-hour flu seven different times. I went from 150 pounds to 125.

The CAT scan revealed nothing and blood tests the same. My doctor was puzzled and told me it was beyond her expertise. She said she would make an appointment for me with another doctor.

Instead of staying home doing nothing and waiting for the time to pass, I took things into my own hands.

I had lost my appetite and was just eating two small meals a day. So, for lunch, I started drinking a complete nutritional drink. I began walking for a half an hour every other day. One morning, after two weeks of my new routine, I woke up feeling free of all my symptoms and I had an appetite. I have now regained my weight and my strength.

While walking near my house one day on the bicycle trail along the San Gabriel River, I saw people speeding past me on their bicycles. Joggers, too, ran past me.

If only they could stop once in a while and smell the sweet odor of blue sage, or see the beauty of the tiny wildflowers, like the chia, or watch the migration of the small painted-lady butterflies, they would, like me, be reminded that it's great to be alive.

— Robert Prado

Carole was in isolation and too weak to leave her hospital bed as she recovered from a stem cell transplant, but not so weak she couldn't benefit from nature's healing powers.

Virtual Nature

I've soared through space to galaxies beyond. I've visited the fuzzy edge of infinity. And now I'm back with an incredible story to tell.

Hold it. Wait a moment. Where on earth did this wild, crazy thought come from? I haven't left the hospital in weeks. How could I have gone anywhere tethered to an IV pole and confined to the isolation of my room?

Perplexed and puzzled, I pondered that intriguing thought for several days. Then the answer came.

One of the most common conditions of being hospitalized is learning how to deal with the fear of pain and the fear of the unknown.

I was told that the hospital television system had a nature channel, which ran continuously with images and music that might help promote healing.

So, for endless hours I watch the most amazing scenes of nature unfold before me. From captivating sunsets to gentle raindrops, the visuals entertain me. I feel the rustling of the wind through the aspen trees, the splashing and invigorating rolling ocean waves, and I bask in the beauty of an enchanting forest.

I am treated to the frolicking of Alaskan bear cubs, and I witness the majestic Canadian geese migrating south for the winter. I see dancing daffodils among mountain wild flowers. I see mighty eagles soaring through wispy clouds. And how can I forget the line of ducks waddling through reeds by the edge of a pond?

But then, when 10 p.m. arrives, the show is suddenly over. No more ducks. No more geese, black bears, gentle rains, babbling creeks, or crashing waves. Has the whole world gone to sleep?

I remember how crushed I was when it first happened. The long night was still before me. How could I endure it with my gnawing worries and fearful thoughts?

Magically, as if I am being transported to another world, the screen goes dark, well almost. Then the real show begins. As I watch, I feel as if I have journeyed to the outer galaxies, and, with a smile on my face, I drift into much-needed slumber.

— Carole Palmquist

Charles Fell was unable to do almost anything. His hands could not grasp a pen, he could not use a computer or hold a telephone, nor could he hold a book to read. But his mind was sharp. While recovering from his bone marrow transplant, he and his wife, Elena, resided in a cottage in the Hope Village. One chance encounter he had while being wheeled around the City of Hope's campus with its colorful plants, shrubs, trees, ponds, and wildlife changed his outlook. Charles memorized his poem, which gave thanks to nature and the generosity of others. His loving wife wrote it down for him.

From the Heart

A squirrel leaps from limb to limb,
Stops and stares at me, and I at him.
After too long a wait
He scatters to the tree's other side,
And, for a while, he hides;
But then, to my surprise,
He peeks out at me, and then again!
This warms my heart and lessens my pain,

And thanks well up inside of me,
To the squirrel, of course, but to others as well:
To those whose names are on the Legacy Wall,
and those who gave us the Walk of Roses,
And the walks of other names.
For the Garden Chapel
And the statue of the Virgin of Guadalupe,
To the City of Hope, its doctors and staff,
And the volunteers they train.
And to my Creator, in whose loving hands I remain.

— Charles F. Fell

Edna sees art in nature and nature in art.

The Master Artist

Whoever used the words "mother" and "nature" in the same sentence got it right. Nature is like a nurturing mother, bringing comfort, inspiring us, giving us a framework of beauty in which to exist. Trees, flowers, water cascading off rocks, the sky when the trees smile after their bath.

When I see a flower in bloom, I feel hopeful.

Maybe God lives in a church, temple, or mosque — I don't know.

But one thing I'm sure of. God the Master Artist created the palette of nature, to nourish and refresh our hopes, our spirits, and our souls.

— Edna Teller

When offered a plethora of venues, Bill decided to, "Make mine nature."

Nature: The Best Medicine

On one end of the bell curve are California's freeways, with cars streaking past, weaving in and out of lanes. On the other end is nature — the mountains on one side, the ocean on the other, with something new to see and marvel at with every step. Where would you rather be?

Throughout my life, I always preferred natural phenomena to manmade civilization. From the beginning of time, man has created the necessities of living. It has been a requirement for survival, I know, but, taken in context, those creations are "fake."

How pleasant is a harmonious walk in the woods, where birds greet your arrival, leaves rustle as nature breathes, and water gurgles its way from rock to rock.

When contrasted to a walk between concrete structures reverberating with the sounds of passing vehicles, cell phones demanding attention, and the cacophony of countless other background noises, there is no contest. No mystery exists in the creation of blacktop and concrete jungles.

Sit in any one of nature's cathedrals and marvel at the complexity, feel the solitude, and heal in the sights and sounds that surround and pacify you. Or wonder at the silence: mountains — rugged and imposing; valleys — green, fertile; deserts — unique and mysterious; oceans — rolling to rhythms all their own. And if the variety of structures wasn't enough, each venue changes constantly with the weather.

As individuals, we are complex and mysterious. Nature is complex and mysterious. What better place to blend in and heal?

— Bill Matteson

Joan's new apartment is where she has wanted to be for a lifetime.

By the Sea

"What makes you love the ocean?" was a question I was asked often over the years.

There was never a logical response. I hadn't thought about it, really, until the weekend my husband was served with our divorce papers, and I felt an overwhelming desire to be beside the sea.

They say a divorce is like a death, and I would have agreed as I sat on the sand, tears streaming down my face, trying to stifle my sobs so I wouldn't attract any attention.

Watching the waves advance and recede was hypnotic, and I found myself growing calmer as time passed. After about an hour, my tears had stopped, and I was ready to face going home again.

When I was diagnosed with cancer, the word I heard and read most often was visualize. "Visualize your cancer as an animal and shoot it down. Visualize the illness and destroy it."

"It doesn't work," I countered.

Wait a minute. Wasn't that what I was doing when I went to the sea? Letting the tide carry my troubles away — far, far away — and return a gentle peace in their place?

The transcendental meditation guru disagreed, but I knew I was right. It's been six years now since my diagnosis, and there have been many healing trips to spend time close to the ocean. It's been a year since I retired and came to live by the sea.

Every morning I look out on the vast expanse of water. Sometimes there are sailboats, sometimes surfers, sometimes only the waves, hurrying to and from the shore.

And always, there is serenity.

— Joan Smith

Even after Dave had been given the news that an infection had invaded his brain and his heart, he turned to nature to help him heal.

The Autumn of Life

The "vegetation" on my heart is called endocarditis. If left unchecked it could damage my heart valves permanently. The spots in my brain are being treated as part of this infection with the hope that it will also respond to this heavy barrage of drugs.

All these twists and turns, of course, were not supposed to happen. Each time we think we have met all the obligations of the current treatment, we encounter a detour. But we continue to persevere.

Here on the central coast of California, the leaves have changed colors and the nights have become chilled. I really enjoy autumn. I think it is the best season of the year. I like to wear soft, wooly sweaters and savor the crisp, clear air.

Autumn also means high school football games, rooting for the home team, turning over the garden to prepare for next year, a cozy, warm crackling fire in the fireplace, and staying close to home, as the nights close in earlier and earlier. Autumn is nature's way of taking a rest after the frenetic pace of summer

Recent events have encouraged me to view my life in much the same way. I believe the time is right to take a rest from the battle with cancer. I want to enjoy the autumn and rejuvenate my mind, body, and spirit for the future. This isn't giving up or throwing in the towel time. Instead, Janis and I see it as an opportunity to take our lives in a more meaningful and positive direction.

I believe I have a better chance of surviving cancer if I am fighting for the joy of living instead of from the fear of dying.

— David Key

It's Your Turn

Write about a place you have found to be healing. Describe its sights and sounds. What does nature do for you or to you when you are there? Is it the activity (boating, fishing, hiking, bird watching) that you enjoy or is it the solitude and escape from city noises? Both?

Is there a place in an urban area that provides you with nature's healing? Tell about how and where this happens. Use the sentences below to help get started.

Jump Start

When I go to ... I always feel ... because ...

Just seeing/hearing ... and ... brings me peace.

During my childhood, I loved going to ... because ...

Keep writing about how nature works its magic on you. When you finish, ask yourself if writing about it also helped bring you peace.

Chapter 21

Lessons Learned

*We may not always realize how some kind word
that's timely spoken may boost the wavering spirit.*
— Joy E. Walker Steward

Throughout life, we all learn valuable lessons — sometimes the hard way through our own mistakes, sometimes through the successes or mistakes of others. Going through a traumatic experience, such as having cancer or being a cancer patient's caregiver or relative, allows us to reflect on what we know and how we learned it.

Much has been written about how having cancer or going through a tragedy or life-threatening illness changes someone. Some people's relationships are deepened and enriched. Ongoing family disputes are often settled as relatives choose the high ground and put their differences aside to help a family member in need.

As with any life experience, learning can take place only if the "student" is ready and willing. If the caregivers, nurses, family members, and patients in my classes are not open to change and growth, they

240

probably would not choose to attend in the first place. So, their reactions and outcomes may not always be typical. But I believe they are serving as role models to others throughout the world.

During the discussion on what life has taught them, I tell students to list 10 lessons they have learned from their experiences with cancer or tragedy and to explain, as appropriate, how they learned them. They work on their lists in class and finish them at home. It takes some thinking for them to fully express what they have learned in a list of only 10 lessons.

At the next session, I read them mine.

I've Learned

1. To recognize love in all its many forms and to cherish it. Unlike some, I have been fortunate to receive it from and give it to: parents, a spouse, family members, my students, friends, and neighbors.

2. To value my health. The body I have is my one and only. I must take care of it and make health and fitness a priority. With all its challenges, this body has taken me to the top of the Eiffel Tower and to the bottom of the Grand Canyon. I owe it respect.

3. The Golden Rule applies to every situation — family, friends, neighbors, cities, and countries.

4. A career is only rewarding when it changes the world for the better. Teaching, to me, is rewarding for that reason.

5. The old saying, "A friend in need is a friend, indeed." couldn't be more true. My friends have helped me conquer many obstacles, cancer being the toughest.

6. The written word is one of the most powerful forces on earth. It can hurt or heal, help or destroy.

7. There is good in the world and there is evil. We need to know the difference. After 9/11, I have witnessed the best and the worst in

humankind.

8. Each generation needs to give back, to sacrifice time and energy to make their family, their town, their world a better place.

9. Cancer is just a word. We will all die of something someday.

10. Humor is essential to health and happiness. It is within our power to choose when to laugh and when to cry.

Healing Words

After cancer, Janet's life couldn't have been more different from her previous one. She wasn't a risk taker and she was often fearful of new experiences. That all changed when she heard the words, "You have cancer."

Life Awakening

It is a rude awakening to hear the doctor say that you have cancer. At first you're in denial. Then you realize that you do, indeed, have cancer and you're going to have to deal with it. I had non-Hodgkin's lymphoma.

The first time it showed up, I went through my chemotherapy treatments fairly well. That put me into remission, thank God. Five months later my cancer returned. I then went through stronger chemotherapy treatments, which put it into remission once again.

At that time my oncologist told me that I would have to undergo a stem cell transplant to keep it from returning. Not much of a choice. Soon after, I checked into the City of Hope for a five-week stay. First on the agenda was for them to take stem cells from me. I would get them back later, my doctors reassured me. I went through many tests and treatments, including total body radiation and heavy doses of chemotherapy prior to getting my stem cells back.

With my transplant complete, I was on the road to recovery. I am thankful my husband and family were with me daily. I am also thankful for the special people who donated platelets for me so I could get stronger. As soon as my blood counts came up, I went home. Here I am, almost eight years later and feeling good. But my life has changed. Life means so much more to me now. As a cancer survivor, here are five life lessons I have learned:

Life is precious. Every day is precious.

I am thankful for my loving family and friends. Enjoy them daily.

Live life in a positive way. Stay away from negative thoughts.

Don't worry about meaningless, petty things. Life is too short.

And, of course, be thankful for good health.

Over the years, I had fears that had prevented me from fully enjoying life. As a cancer survivor, I look at life differently. I have conquered those fears and added fun and great enjoyment to my life.

— Janet Gray

(Following this writing, Janet's husband and her mother died within two month's time. Although fragile, Janet is still attending Writing for Wellness classes and volunteering at City of Hope. In addition, she and her daughter colorfully hand painted 250 baseball hats and presented them to hospitalized cancer patients.)

When Esteban came to class, he looked weak, sad, and very young. He was a college student in his early 20s and had just undergone a bone marrow transplant. Some of the BMT survivors in class saw his pain and immediately took him under their wings. Christine went on a walk with him through the Japanese Garden on campus, Bill took him fishing, Robin took him to dinner and medical appointments, and Anna served as his soft shoulder, hearing him out and cheering him up. Over time, he looked stronger, happier, and older. In Esteban's own words he explains.

Lessons from Hard Times

I'm 24, a native of Colombia. My only sister Carolina Jaramillo was a perfect match for my bone marrow transplant. I can honestly say it was the power of writing that helped me get through everything little by little (baby steps). This is the first writing I ever did in Writing for Wellness class although I came to class many times and listened to writings of others. I was just too sad, too upset to write about what I was going through. Then, once I began to put my thoughts down, I learned that writing had become very good medicine.

As I listened to the rain on a Saturday night, it made me homesick as I thought about the hard times that I had this year. As I listened to the rain it made me realize that I have actually been a brave and courageous man by facing this hurdle with lots of patience and mental strength. But it was something I had to learn through time.

Now, today I know there is a God who not only saves but cures. I know this by the fact that He allowed my only sibling to be the tool to cure my cancer. I thank City of Hope and feel very fortunate to be here and feel very pleased with everyone who has been there for me through good and bad times.

To this day I'm struggling with the emotional and psychological part of my ordeal. Trust me, it hasn't been easy. The way I feel is that something was taken away from me at this early part of my life and I have to go through a process to emotionally feel better about the big obstacle that I overcame.

It's been five months since my bone marrow transplant and I thought the hardest part would recovering physically. That part was hard, don't get me wrong. But now I think I'm facing another process (depression and anxiety) and I really need my two new best friends, Time and Patience, to help me through it. Even though I just turned 24, I'm sure the whole experience has made me grow up in every aspect of my life. I believe things are done for a reason and God chooses the toughest ones to face the big obstacles. I'm sure God had a purpose in my life that little by little He'll guide me to where He wants me to be.

— Esteban Jaramillo

(Esteban completed training to become a phlebotomist and is working at a local hospital. He wants to continue in the medical field in order to "give back" to others.)

Joy's poem reflects a new philosophy gained through dealing with her cancer.

Each One Helping Each One

We are all dying, this human race.
We've all been prescribed, a time and place.
Living or dying, we all blaze a trail.
For those who come after, we each tell a tale.
Even my struggles may strengthen another,
A few paces behind me, a sister or brother.
The knowledge I gain as I fight for my health,
When shared with others, brings me much wealth.
And the sister before me, who's losing the fight,
Still walks with dignity and gives me insight,
Into how I should live, 'til it's my time to go,
Each one helping each one, to soften the blow.
I hope when I'm gone, that the trail I have blazed,
Will have for some traveler, a smoother path paved.

— Joy E. Walker Steward

Rick's lessons reflect strong values and a sense of humor.

Life Lessons

1. General human nature doesn't change, but people do transform throughout their lives. The explosion of marriages and of divorce rates may be the earmark of the post-Christian era. Today's church wedding ceremony is mostly the kickoff for an expensive coming-out party.

2. Women denied careers during their childbearing years seek job fulfillment at a time when they should be enjoying the reflective years. Greener grasses come at a price.

3. If one gets caught up in politics, one learns quickly that "spin" degenerates the intellect along with one's moral fiber. Fast talkers are viewed as more credible, and sound bites feed mob psychology.

4. If you cannot control negatives, change the way you think about them, and keep healthy within. Mothers-in-law and crazy neighbors come to mind.

5. The best medications come from selecting with care what we choose to put into our mouths.

6. The sooner we learn that life presents us with a never-ending series of challenges, the more comfortable we'll be with chaos. Raising kids comes to mind.

7. People of the world rarely self-regulate over time. Unfortunately, justice tends toward the interest of the stronger.

8. While exercise may regulate our inner chaos, it also triggers compulsive propensities.

9. You may not like them but one always has choices.

10. Faith in God is the ultimate fallback position. Still, it takes periodic reminders to affirm that one basic truth.

— Rick Myers

I have known Buddy for 45 years. My husband Bob and her son, Stefan, have been best friends since Bob was 12. Buddy, a retired New York City teacher, has been interested in art since taking oil-painting classes in Brooklyn in the 1950s. When she and her husband, Sam, moved to California, she continued taking classes.

Her teachers and others who viewed her work consistently said she had a unique gift. At age 68, she began studying ceramics, but also wanted to learn Chinese brush painting to decorate her ceramic pieces. She has continued to study brush painting for 13 years. She has won awards for her work and has traveled twice with her teacher and classmates to China. Her life seemed good until one day when she felt a strange pain in her side.

A Lesson for the Teacher

I had been told by a gastroenterologist that there was nothing wrong with me, that my right side bothered me because I was merely shrinking with age. I didn't need a colonoscopy, he reassured me.

My regular doctor and I didn't like that explanation and he insisted that I undergo a colonoscopy. The test revealed two cancerous tumors in my colon. To me, at my age (91), it meant the end. I was devastated and scared. However, I decided to have the surgery.

Wonder of wonders, the surgeon took out a piece of my colon that contained the tumors and left me in great condition — no radiation needed. I had caught it in time before the tumors grew or spread.

The lesson? It's good to listen to what your body tells you.

— Buddy Steinberg

(Now that Buddy's cancer is gone, she continues brush painting and is planning another trip to China.)

Even for someone in his 20s, Jeff's lessons, learned through his mother's battle with lung cancer, may last him a lifetime.

Hard Lessons

I have learned to appreciate the moments I have with my mother, even the ones that once annoyed me. Despite the initial pain it has caused, I learned that I have to be less selfish about my time.

I have learned that no matter how much I want to believe that these kinds of things happen to "other people," my family is also at risk.

I have gained a better understanding of the treatment options involved with cancer, and how to recognize the progression of the pathology.

I now realize that this strong woman who packs more punch into her 5 foot 2 frame than I thought possible is also capable of being just as scared as I am.

However, I also learned that my mother, even when faced with the prospect of death, can still be just as strong as I have always known.

— Jeff Howe

After her mother, movie producer Linda Bergman, was diagnosed with leukemia, Sarah learned valuable lessons that she still remembers.

A Life Lesson

I was 16. My mother's leukemia diagnosis couldn't have come at a more challenging time personally. I was in the midst of raging hormonal imbalance. I had separating parents, social anxiety, college applications due, and an all-around, good-old revolutionary adolescent attitude.

The great mystery of life was unfolding at an already alarming rate, and to have my mother's possible death thrown into the mix was, well, inconvenient and utterly overwhelming.

I was resentful that this crisis was upon us. Cancer is not pretty. The fear of death is not comfortable. It seemed as though every second of the day I was struggling to find a way to not feel afraid, searching tirelessly for ways to cope with or understand this difficult time.

I wondered if running away was my answer. I wondered if these healers that were coming to our house could brew the right potion to bring my mother back into herself and back to us.

I even wondered if death was the answer. If she just died and her pain went away, could my suffering go away, too?

Such are the questions we ask in the face of fear.

I was surviving. Sometimes I was a supportive daughter who would give my mom manicures and replenish the flowers by her bed, showing up with hope and the zest for life. Sometimes I was a depleted, helpless, and angry 16 year old who wanted to get as far from home as possible.

The stakes were very high in this time of desperation. I was desperate to be with her, and desperate to be away from her. I needed her to live and to be healthy so that I could be a young girl who was excited to go to her prom.

In the process of surviving, there are endless surprises. You think everything is hopeless. Then on a street corner, you see a baby smile and all of a sudden life is a blessing again. For me a surprise came in what at the time was a very common circumstance in my household, my mom was lying in bed.

One day, after school, I went upstairs to her room where she was resting. I looked at her. There was a particular peace about her. There seemed to be a kind of release and stillness in her being.

For the first time since her diagnosis, I felt completely at peace and okay with what was. I felt like I got a taste of what it would be like for my mom to let go. I felt relief. In that moment, she was at peace, I was at peace, and I was grateful.

Luckily, my unbelievably wonderful mother is still with us, and we are blessed to be able to continue this abundant life together.

What I learned from that moment at her bedside is that peace is always available to us. Life is hard, but when those moments of peace come, take them, hold them, breathe into them, cherish them.

When death comes to a loved one, I hope to be able to feel the reverberations of that moment by her bedside.

What I have also learned is that cancer can be messy. Sickness can breed doubt and dark thoughts, but it is not our job to judge ourselves in the face of something real and scary. It is our job to be present and to keep hope alive.

— **Sarah Bergman**

It's Your Turn

What lessons have you learned so far in your life? Make a list of five to ten. Explain in a few words how you learned these lessons. What lessons would you like your children or friends to learn from your mistakes? Use the sentences below if you need help getting started.

Jump Start

The most important lesson I learned about (people, money, my goals) was ...

I learned the hard way that ...

I would like to tell my children or friends to always ...

I wish my parents had told me ...

Chapter 22

Your Story/Your Legacy

Your character is your legacy.

— Doug Wilkey

The word legacy can mean many different things to many people. It might be something you created, a scholarship or grant to continue what you started or to give back to a favorite cause or institution. Or it might be simply a way of thinking you hope will endure after you are gone. When I ask students to write about what legacy they would like to leave behind, what results comes from as many different perspectives as there are people in the class. Some want to write, paint, sculpt, sew, build, or compose. They want to leave something tangible. Others want to change lives, attitudes, the direction of the country or world — important, although not as immediately visible.

Nothing says you can't do all of the above. But it has been my experience that if you want to leave your family something priceless, you might consider starting with the written word.

First answer this. What would you give for a hand-written, scribbled, but legible story full of misspelled words on yellowed paper? Someone on eBay might buy it sight unseen. Who knows if it would go for one dollar or a thousand?

But what if that story were written by your great, great grandfather about his life?

Every person's story is unique and has value. The time, the places, and the circumstances combine to allow the reader, even centuries later, to live and relive what an ancestor did, felt, thought, and may have died for.

Even their day-to-day activities would be compelling to read.

I was fortunate to have the opportunity to read such a story into a tape recorder for a man I met at the YMCA where I go to swim and attend water aerobics every weekday morning.

Sidney was 90 years old and very witty. He was also blind. I was surprised to learn that for several years he had come to the Y each morning to exercise and swim. He joked with all of us who, along with him, were trying to keep our aging bodies from giving up on us. Each day when he greeted his fellow exercisers, he'd say with a completely straight face, "You look great!"

One day he mentioned that he had in his possession a diary written by one of his ancestors. It was about his experience with the handcart Mormon pioneers who had walked from Nauvoo, Illinois, starting in 1847 pulling their belongings on carts along the 1,300-mile journey to the Salt Lake Valley.

Sidney had read the diary many times before losing his sight and longed to read it again. I was interested in learning more about the story and I also liked Sidney. I told him I would read the diary into a tape recorder for him so he could play the tape whenever he wished. It only took me a few hours.

He was delighted. But, as with so many gestures like this, I was the one who benefited most.

The story of those courageous pioneers who braved political and religious persecution, along with the elements, was fascinating. His uncle had merely recorded their day-to-day struggles, but, in doing so, he also told the story of his lifetime. We learned about their lack of food and clothing, we learned about those who died in childbirth or from diseases, and we learned that when they arrived, they believed they had come to the promised land.

Over the years, Sidney would talk to me about the diary and thank me for taping it. I thanked him for the privilege.

For the last ten years I have taught seminars in the Los Angeles area for women's groups, historical societies, and teacher groups on the subject, "Writing Your Own Story" and "Writing Your Family's History." I volunteer to do this because I love to see people get excited about writing and then follow through and actually do it.

People seem fascinated with talking about writing, but when it gets down to doing it, well, that's another story. I tell students in my classes, "There are two kinds of people — those who like to talk about writing and those who actually DO it. You are going to be in the latter category!"

To make sure that happens I distribute paper and pencils and, after just a short introduction, I give them instructions on how to begin.

In Writing for Wellness, students are often highly motivated to tell their stories. After all, they don't know how long they have left on earth and they want to leave their thoughts and their feelings behind.

Here are some steps to get you started:

1. Give a brief family background statement. Don't start 100 years ago with who married whom. It will sound like the Book of Genesis with all of its "begats." You may get bored and never finish the story. Whoever picks it up might have the same reaction.

2. Instead, write a short summary of your own life.

3. Focus on meaningful events in your life. You cannot possibly tell nor would anyone want to read every detail of every day of your life.

Therefore, organize your ideas into significant segments such as: my family and how we interacted; school(s); a holiday I'll never forget; teachers; friends; the first time I earned money; career; how I felt about my family and my role in it.

4. Also include categories such as: junior high; high school; college; first date; first love; lasting love; hard times; deaths in the family; favorite relative; craziest relative; marriage; divorce (Hey, it happens!); first child, next child; successes, successes of the children; those teenage years; romantic moments; humorous memories; retirement; grandchildren; great grandchildren; best and worst trips and vacations; religion; politics; world events; and, finally, how you would like to be remembered.

5. Use a three ring binder or computer folders with these headings and you will be all set. You don't have to write your story in chronological order. When a certain mood strikes and you remember something, get out your notebook and find the proper chapter for your story of the day.

Or turn on your computer and keyboard in those memories. Feedback I get indicates this method seems to work. Writing your family history sounds overwhelming. Writing a simple story of one event in your life sounds like much more fun. Try it.

Healing Words

Students in my classes are of all different ages. The youngest I have had was 15. The oldest have been in their 90s. The common ground for most is cancer or another life-changing condition that motivates many to write. Some, especially the younger students, prefer to write nostalgic stories, remembering times before their disease changed the direction of their lives. Even the idea of a legacy is difficult for them to grasp. But in writing about their happy times, they are creating a legacy just the same.

Others, the older students in most cases, want their children and grandchildren to know how hard life was during depression or recession years or before computers were invented. Still others, those who have served in wars, want to let the young people in their lives know what sacrifices were made to make our country free. Conversely, those who witnessed terrible events want to warn their grandchildren about the "glories" of war and urge them to try to make the world a more peaceful, forgiving place.

Here are some of the varied writings that resulted from the family history/legacy assignment.

Not knowing if she will survive her cancer, Christine, at age 31, says she has more questions than answers about the legacy she wants to leave behind. First, she wants to define what a legacy means to her. Next, she asks the readers to examine their lives through answering a series of questions she poses.

My Legacy? Ultimately our greatest and deepest desire is to give a gift to this world before we leave. This legacy may be in the form of building a library, writing a song, or perhaps bearing a child. This is proof that at our core, we love one another. We cannot feel satisfied with the life we have lived until we have given away the greatest part of ourselves. My poem asks the questions. Only you have the answers.

What Will You Bring?

What will you help bring into this world?
Music? Laughter? Perhaps a child?
What will your hands create?

What will your voice carry?

What will you leave behind?

What will you give to the future?

How will you share with the present?

Who will you love?

What good will you make with this life?

How will you make God manifest?

Whose souls will you teach?

Whose heart will you save?

What will you bring into this world, this living life?

What will you give?

Your talent? Your time? Your own life?

What beauty will you create while you are here?

What wondrous something will you be the vessel for?

What will you put on this earth, create in this universe,

Before you leave us?

— Christine Pechera

Carole, in the midst of preparing for a double stem cell transplant to stop multiple myeloma, writes about reading her mother's autobiography, and, in doing so leaves her own legacy.

Mirrored Legacy

Her nickname was Attila the Hun, a name she both despised and embraced. Outwardly, she appeared to be a mild-mannered, conforming lady. She dressed conservatively and could always be found wearing her signature "grandma" white wig and her triple strand of pearls.

For 85 years, my mother could boast that she had never been sick a day in her life. She managed to dodge most physical afflictions — no cancer, diabetes, heart ailments, arthritis, or even allergies. She lived a long life despite bending the "rules." She cooked with plenty of fats and real mayonnaise, and she relished her desserts — the ones loaded with old-fashioned calories. And, instead of exercising, she much preferred to exercise her vocal chords on the telephone.

She also refused to wear seatbelts in the car and, when reminded it was the law, would say, "It goes against my freedom!"

Despite this, my mother was a God-fearing, law-abiding citizen in every other way. She never indulged in any vices. She never drank, smoked, gambled, danced, or used profanity. Mom's life seemed like a bowl of cherries. Until that one morning.

Reaching for a large bottle of cranberry juice, she lost her balance and lay on the floor with a broken hip. She died five months later.

I am writing this on Mother's Day, a time for reflection, a time for reverence, and a time for respect for mothers. She was born on May 10, often celebrated as Mother's Day.

I'm drawn to contemplate the meaning of her life as I sit here at her command post, a cushy green armchair where she spent hours of her time. I see her well-used phone covered with smudge marks. I gaze out her picture window overlooking her front yard.

On the opposite wall, I see her family gallery of photos, which includes her four children, their spouses, 12 grandchildren, and one great-grandchild.

I open a book, her autobiography, a book painstakingly written over a period of a year. I see what a gift she left as she struggled to answer those penetrating questions about her life as a child and young adult. I think about her spirit of determination.

As I read, I see her in a new way. I remember how she talked about her early life in America. Born to Norwegian immigrants, she shared in her family's struggles of survival in their new country.

She writes about the trauma she experienced when she was three and her father suddenly died, leaving a hole that could be not filled throughout her life. The most devastating part was that her father's name was never mentioned again.

Work was a priority as the weight of being the sole breadwinner now shifted to her mother's shoulders.

There was no time for grief, no Dr. Phil and no Dr. Laura. This was true Norwegian grit. When my mother complained about anything, her mother would say, "Work hard and you'll feel better."

Time has come to accept and embrace that same spirit of Attila that resides in me.

It's as if I've been peering into a mirror. For I see the same traits. I have to admit that I am also head strong, impetuous, stubborn, and determined. I am my mother's daughter. As I begin to understand her, I find the comfort of forgiveness. I find room to accept my own frailties and the courage to channel this Norwegian spirit as I prepare to fight the battles ahead.

— **Carole Palmquist**

Edna finds the entire idea of leaving a legacy somewhat puzzling.

Living My Legacy

Pardon me, but have you seen my legacy?

It was here just a minute ago. Now it's gone, and I don't know when it'll be back. Let me know if it contacts you, ok?

Or, maybe I should post a flyer on the bulletin board at the supermarket: "Lost, one legacy. Still in development, fragile when exposed to life's hardships. Often seen in the company of an ego. If found, notify Self."

Maybe I'm being more than a bit facetious, but really, thinking about one's legacy can be daunting. For one thing, legacy usually implies that you have departed from this earthly realm, and I'm not sure I want to contemplate that certainty in any depth.

Also, the word connotes something important or imposing, like a hospital wing or university endowment.

In fact, Webster's defines legacy both as "a gift by will especially of money or other personal property" and "something transmitted by or received from an ancestor or predecessor or from the past." Both definitions imply a transfer of something valuable.

It got me thinking about the concept of a legacy, and what that means for me personally. I don't expect to leave my family millions of dollars, and my personal possessions, while valuable to me, will not trigger an important estate sale at Sotheby's. So, I ask myself, will I leave a legacy at all? How will I be remembered? The thoughts are more than a little disturbing. I talked to good friends, and mulled over the issue some more.

After a few days, I came to a conclusion that surprised and pleased me, because it was both simple and spiritually satisfying.

If you believe, as Einstein did, that all matter is energy and that it is constantly moving, then all of our actions have energetic consequences. We can manifest both positive and negative energy, and it can be a conscious choice.

I have chosen to leave a legacy not only to my friends and family, but also to our global family on this Earth. I can make a difference every day in my interactions with other people, those I know and those I do not know. I can smile at the mail clerk at the post office and let her know what a good job she does. I can let the frazzled mother go through the supermarket check stand before me. I can make someone's day with a smile or a cheery, "Good morning!"

The positive energy passes to others, who pass it on again, and so it goes.

I like this legacy. It makes sense to me. It doesn't require money or fame, just a desire to change the world for the better, one person at a time.

I'm going for it.

— **Edna Teller**

Joy's family history story bridges two countries.

A Tribute to Mama

I believe the best tribute a person can give to their mother is to emulate her good example, forgive her weaknesses, and learn what not to do. Each generation would be better than the previous one if we set ourselves to do that.

Mama was a Type-A personality and the chip did not fall far from the block. Kevin Lehman, in his birth order book, points out that all firstborns are perfectionists. We are the ones our parents practiced on the hardest.

An industrious, resourceful woman, Mama knew how to make a little go a long way. That trait has served me well in my fixed-income status as a single parent. "Cleanliness is next to Godliness" was one of her favorite sayings. "If you go out all dressed up and pretty and your house is a mess, you are going to be embarrassed if something happens to you and a stranger has to bring you home."

We lived much of our lives in tenement houses in Kingston, Jamaica, before coming to this country. Showers and toilets were shared, and Mama, aware of all the germs her children might pick up, never allowed us to go barefoot.

She was forever scrubbing, scouring, and sanitizing. She loved a clean, orderly house and so do I. Mama's speech was as clean as her person. Mama had class. She was a lady with never a cuss word on her lips. She did not have more than a sixth-grade education but she was very polished in her demeanor. She taught her children to read using the King James Bible. Character, she taught us, was what you did when no one but God was looking.

— Joy E. Walker Steward

Linda, a breast cancer survivor herself who has worked at City of Hope for eight years, wrote about another patient who formed a foundation to provide minority women with low-cost mammograms and information about detection and prevention, leaving a unique legacy.

Hattie Anderson's Legacy

According to Rita Dove, America's first Black Poet Laureate, "Courage has nothing to do with our determination to be great. It has to do with what we decide in that moment when we are called upon."

Hattie decided when she was called upon not only to be more, but to do more. And she did so up until her last earthly breath. After Hattie was initially diagnosed with breast cancer in 1993, she made a conscious decision to refocus her energies. She had at one time been heavily involved in political fundraising.

Then she launched a campaign to bring breast cancer awareness to under-served women in Los Angeles. She teamed with the City of Hope for a special outreach effort to minority women providing them with free breast cancer education workshops.

Suffering from an extremely aggressive form of cancer that returned three times, Hattie often said, "You have to stop worrying about dying so you can live."

She roamed the hallways at the medical center looking for that one person who needed her most. She could always tell who they were —

the scared, the uncertain, the exhausted.

Hattie would lift them up in a way no one else could. She offered her shoulder to lean on and a heart as wide as a mile, almost as wide as her smile.

Her presence has lingered in the gardens and hallways she loved and watched over. Her legacy of service, advocacy, compassion, and love will live on in the hearts of staff, patients, and volunteers that she so deeply touched. She was my hero.

I was honored to read the following poem at the celebration of Hattie's life.

New Sunrise

She lay to rest when the moon was full,
A life abundant and rich and deep.
Her measure declared by Love all around,
Comfort covered as she went to sleep.
Peace fell on her as sunset approached,
Her new sunrise awaits.
She will carry on her glorious call,
Inspiration at the Gate.

— Linda Baginski

It's Your Turn

Writing your story, the story of a favorite family member, or one about an important person in your life is probably one of the most significant activities you can accomplish. And, with a few shortcuts used by professional writers, you may find it is not only enjoyable, but easy.

When writing about your own life's story or even writing about a political issue or something you want to comment on that was printed in the newspaper, simply use the very first words in your writing to indicate your topic. This will organize the piece and start the logical flow of words.

Example: "My first teacher was..." or "Stem cell research should (or should not) be funded because..."

This technique gets you started right away and from there, you just need to explain yourself, giving the facts to back up your first few words.

Writing professionals call this an "umbrella" statement. Picture an umbrella as having three parts — the cloth top, the pole that holds up the top, and, on the old-fashioned umbrellas, a u-shaped handle. The umbrella statement "covers" the subject. Example: "My aunt Martha almost ruined Christmas one year..." This statement tells everyone what you are writing about and what to expect next. Don't go off on a tangent and start saying how you never liked her son, Bill, either.

Stick to one subject, the one covered by your umbrella statement. As you review the writings in the *Healing Words* section of this chapter, notice how the writers stay on the topic.

Jump Start

These easy-to-use writing "starters" will help you begin to tell stories of your own life or those about your family's history, assisting as you leave your own legacy.

My (Uncle John) was the kindest (craziest) of all of my relatives because ...

A Thanksgiving I'll never forget was when ...

You have your "umbrella statements." Now hold up your own story with a pole of memories.

Chapter 23

Happy Days Are Near Again

Only I can make the sun shine again after a long season of rain.

— Joy. E. Walker Steward

As you emerge from the darkness of pain and fear, there will come a day when the sun rises and lights up your room. The people who were only shadows before come into focus. Instead of living in a microcosm of the world — your hospital room — you return to the real one with all of its defects and promises.

Those around you may notice physical changes. Your color is better, they tell you. You seem to have more energy, others add.

But you, yourself, know that nothing will ever be the same again. Your experience has forever changed your outlook, your expectations, and your goals.

Friends, family, your house — even your car look especially welcome as you leave the confines of the medical world to delve into a new one, one full of hope and promise. When your pet greets you at your front door, your emotions spill out. You were missed. Your dog or cat noticed and came to you for reassurance that you'll never leave again.

You may even want to get back to work too soon. Deep down, you may try to prove to yourself that you never really had cancer, that you are stronger than anyone around you, and that you can work 18 hours a day. You may even do that for a while. A lot of us have.

Neighbors and colleagues at work may seek you out and want to talk to you. By coming home and returning to work and the routines you once followed, you are reassuring them that they, too, are back to normal. They don't have to deal with their own mortality right now. Thank goodness for that. Everyone around you thinks they can see how you've changed, how you've come through this. Only you really know that light is starting to fill your day.

Healing Words

Linda Bergman's son, Adam was 13 at the time of his mother's diagnosis. He writes about how their family experienced disbelief, anguish, and fear, and then together, beat Linda's cancer.

As Powerless as Cancer

Cancer is powerless. As strong and painful as it is on one end, it is equally weak and flimsy at the other.

As a child, cancer is your worst nightmare. You imagine the day that one of your parents gets it, and that day is the end of the world. So like a child, when I found out that my mother had been diagnosed with leukemia, I panicked like a child.

I imagined my life with only my father and my sister, and everything fell apart in my imaginary world. At the time, though, I had no idea how weak cancer really was. I had no idea that cancer could actually make a family better. And I had no idea how strong my mother was.

I watched cancer come into my house and try to break apart my family. I watched it creep inside my father and sister, I felt it inside me, and I watched it try to kill my mother.

But I also saw four human beings triumph over it in a way that can't be described by words. I saw a woman defy all the odds. I saw a woman with an expiration date muster more power than any cancer could ever bestow upon her. I watched a family come together to do the unthinkable. We beat cancer.

So we proved that cancer is powerless. We have a magnet on our refrigerator that helps put into words what I saw in my house when cancer tried to come in. To quote it,

"What cancer cannot do: It cannot cripple love; it cannot shatter hope; it cannot corrode faith; it cannot destroy peace; it cannot kill friendship; it cannot suppress memories; it cannot silence courage; it cannot invade the soul; it cannot steal eternal life; it cannot conquer the spirit." (Unknown).

— **Adam Bergman**

As a class assignment, Rick had the choice of writing about either the best of times or the worst of times in his son's fight with cancer. He wrote the following:

Best of Times

The day my son, Rick, attended his first City of Hope anniversary celebration for bone marrow transplant survivors, my mind flashed back to some of the many threatening episodes that we sweated through in his treatment — treatments that now seem to have occurred years ago and in a different world.

But on that celebratory day, the son that I knew — reserved, acutely observant of others, cautious in acceptance of the unknown in humans and in events, fragile still but wearing his one-year anniversary pin on his belt rather than his lapel — looked out with a fresh recognition at the gathering of kindred souls who had bled as he had, fallen as he had, each heroic, each restored as God had willed. My son was one of them.

My feeling as an outsider was that of watching war veterans acknowledge one another — reluctant to share completely unless with an inmate — beyond the understanding of those who only stood and waited, but served still.

The gradations of human experience opened wider to those who celebrated that special day. Did it confer immunity to future ordeals? Or rather cause them to recoil in defense, playing carefully with what is left lest it be snatched up as quickly as a losing casino bet?

My observation was that their conversations had come at a profound cost, that of fast-forwarding their lives to the mindset of one far more mature, and one who reflects backward as much as forward. A portion of the wonder of life is excised by those who've tasted the outcome — a movie viewed by one who's read the book.

Yet, the faces I saw reflected a joy of deliverance and of celebration, hardly victims, more like heroes.

— Rick Myers

Imagine a year without the change of seasons — no spring, summer, or fall — only winter for 12 months straight. This was the type of year that just ended for Carole. A black cloud had taken up permanent residence over her as she struggled with constant treatments and coped with personal grief and loss. Still, throughout her ordeal, she felt she needed to write, and in the process her seasons changed.

Spring

When I hear Vivaldi's masterpiece Spring march across my radio at 5:30 a.m., I know this day is destined to be extraordinary.

My heart leaps with joy as I realize that my cold, bleak winter of loss and grief is finally departing. Tearfully, I marvel at the thought that I actually have survived the past year. I am alive! I really am alive!

Then I realize what has sustained me through this dreadful winter-like experience is my writing. I think about all that I have written and I am comforted by re-reading my poems and prose. As I reminisce, I realize that when I started to write, I had no idea what I was doing or why. I only knew that something inside me was compelling, no commanding, me to express these thoughts. I recall how many times early in the morning I would awaken and write with an unrelenting fervor without regard to direction or result.

I laugh out loud at the thought of becoming a writer. After all, I had always dreaded that activity more than anything else in the world. It was sheer torture for me. I remember the excruciating pain I suffered from writer's block — more like writer's hysteria to be precise. And now, I had been writing this year as if my life depended upon it.

I think about how I first began. Again, I chuckle when I realize that indeed my subconscious mind actually tricked me into it. At first, I just would play with words on a small spiral tablet kept with me at all times. I compiled word lists. I had no problem making them since I had plenty of experience making grocery lists and "honey-do" lists over the years.

For hours, I would think of words and then become excited when I discovered yet another one to add to my list. One list was for the colors. "Black" eventually was the subject of my first poem. Since then, I have discovered that black psychologically represents the cancer in my body. That revelation still sends shivers throughout my being.

Rereading my works breathes life into my weary soul. I can scarcely contain the joy and the wonderment I feel that while my life seemed laced with heavy grief, my spirit had been kept alive. Writing had been my lifeline.

— Carole Palmquist

As a survivor, Marilyn finds she is grateful for things other people usually take for granted.

A Grateful Day

Good morning, God.
Thank you that I can wake up,
that I can look up.
Thank you that I can sit up,
that I can get up.
Thank you that I can stand up,
that I can stay up.
Thank you that I can reach up,
open up, and,
choose to be up.
Finally, at the end of the day,
Thank you that I can kneel down,
and then lie down,
to rest through the night
in your love and care.
Good night, God.

— Marilyn Butler

Jeff's mother's lung cancer was bringing the family closer and making them more positive day by day.

A Warm and Safe House

I don't know if I'm simply seeing what I want to see, but since my mother was diagnosed with lung cancer, there aren't the normal rounds of bickering and fighting that go on in any family. I personally think that there just isn't a need for it anymore. There is something more important. Why waste time arguing?

My parents have always been close, and my mom's cancer hasn't changed that a great deal. But what it has done is make my parents realize that the life they wanted to have together — now that we children are all gone — has to start now.

It's sad in a way. My father says he feels a little cheated. My parents worked all their adult lives to raise children, knowing that eventually they would be together again, alone. Now that might be taken from them.

So every moment is cherished. We don't sit around wondering if this will be the last time we have a good day, but we do have fun with one another.

My parents' home has become more welcoming, a place where everyone can feel safe, where the word "cancer" doesn't have to be acknowledged every day. It's there, but so are the dinners and movies in front of the fire.

My family has turned Thanksgiving into a day when we really are thankful for what we have, not just thankful that my nieces haven't spilled anything on the good tablecloth. Christmas holds more meaning, too, with family members and friends making that extra effort to stop by. Friends and family members have become closer emotionally. This closeness actually created healthy changes in the way lives are lived. Some (though sadly not all) have quit smoking completely, or have mitigated their smoking around my mom. This is an example of how we have all made the decision to create a comfortable, loving atmosphere where we can all feel safe.

— Jeff Howe

Linda, a ten-year breast cancer survivor is coordinator for the "Pink Links" support group for breast cancer survivors. Below she writes to the sisterhood created by breast cancer.

The Women We Are

The women we are,
the stitch and the scar,
missing pieces and parts,
but never our hearts.
Unbreakable us.

Potions of red
took toll on our heads.
Connected by fate,
was it early or late?
Unshakeable us.

Scanned and glowing,
our enemies showing.
Singed and seared,
blistered by fear,
but never alone.

For the women we are,
bodies skewed, dreams ajar,
shelters the girl inside,
who can't run and hide.
Who will be saved?
Oh, you must be so brave.

Sorority of souls,
what now is our role?
To embrace the day,
lift out of the gray.
Hold her hands when they shake
with bonds that won't break.
Remarkable us.

For the women we are,
see more clearly by far.
Touch softer knowing,
let tears go flowing.
Listen closer, deeper,
each other's keeper.

For the women we are,
raise higher the bar.
Dig deeper,
love fuller,
measure longer the ruler.
Undeniable us!

— **Linda Baginski**

Though her death was a possible, if not likely outcome, during the days prior to her first bone marrow transplant, Christine wrote in her journal about her prediction — to have a positive result.

Serenity

Tonight I am alone. I choose to be. It will be the last time in a long time when I will be completely by myself and I want this time alone with my thoughts. The next few weeks will decide whether I shall live or die, and if I am going to live a long and healthy life or a gloriously poetic short one.

Tears come easily to me now. I never used to cry in front of people. Now I do all the time.

I am so thankful for all of the close intimate relationships I have, but I also celebrate my freedom to explore and discover the beauty of other human beings.

This all has a purpose. This is bringing everything into balance. There will be prosperity, love, friendship, and success in that balance of polarities.

There will be a return to the natural state of things and all these terrible dramas and events will cancel each other out until there is the serenity and contentedness of effortless balance.

— Christine Pechera

(Christine had just celebrated the two-year anniversary of her bone marrow transplant when she was told it was beginning to fail. Because she is a Filipina, she needed someone of Filipino ethnicity as a donor. Her family members are not viable matches for her. Her classmates, friends, and family members spread the word throughout Los Angeles and on the Internet for those in the Filipino community to be tested. Christine appeared on local and national television news programs to appeal for a donor. She also set up a website that was visited by thousands of people who were trying to save her. Ultimately, she had to proceed with a 50% match, one that gave her less than a 50-50 chance at life. After more than 100 days on the City of Hope campus and many touch-and-go medical crises, she is alive, home, and thriving. Love, prayers, and science were on her side.)

It's Your Turn

After almost any crisis in life, there will be those who see it in a positive light while others view it darkly and never fully recover from its effects. There are those who will learn from it and strive to light the way for others. Where do you want to be? How will writing help you?

Write about where you want to see yourself six months from now, a year from now. How will you be different? To help start your words flowing, use one or all of the sentences below.

Jump Start

Six months from now, I hope to be ...

I am going to work on being ... so that a year from today, I ...

I hope I can always ...

Remember hope is contagious.

Part IV

Compassionate Outcomes

Chapter 24

Family Matters

Mama cared about people and taught me to treat everyone with respect, regardless of his or her status in life.

— Joy E. Walker Steward

As part of one lesson, I ask students to think about a family incident or story that has been on their minds. Some of their stories deal with conflicts that came with the trials and frustrations of cancer diagnosis and treatment. I often tell about the son of one of my closest friends who said he felt it was "too depressing" to visit his father in the hospital where he was battling cancer. When the father recovered, their relationship had been badly, if not irreparably, damaged.

Some class members write as parents who are trying to be brave for children who are cancer patients. Others write as the children trying to cope with the reversal of their roles as caregivers for parents with cancer or other serious diseases.

Other stories recall positive and memorable events from their

277

childhood during which a particular relative served as a role model. To get class members started thinking about family matters, I usually read them an article I wrote about my grandmother, Nana.

A Clean Sweep

On New Year's Day, I always think of my grandmother, Gertrude Lynn Bolger, a woman who always wore flower-print dresses, smelled like wonderful bath powder, and always kept the cleanest house on the block. She prepared each day's meals with fresh vegetables grown in her own garden, or in winter, lovingly preserved ones from her home-canning pantry. She washed clothes in her basement using a wringer washer and hung out the heavy bed sheets to dry on outside clotheslines, even in the bitter Colorado winters. She never owned a clothes dryer, even when everyone else in the family did.

Nana, as I called her, didn't need to go to the gym to stay in shape. She was never overweight, she lived until she was 93, and, importantly, she knew how to use a broom.

It was always late in the year when my grandmother bought a new broom.

Nana was from Pennsylvania, Irish-Catholic stock, and did almost everything in an orderly, deliberate way. And after Thanksgiving was always her broom-buying time.

Her broom had to be of the large natural straw variety, with a sturdy wooden handle, one that would do good service and last an entire year. She would shop for it and carefully examine the straw to be sure it would hold up under pressure.

She never used her new broom until New Year's Day.

When I grew up in Colorado Springs, it was not unusual to see women wearing aprons over their housedresses as they swept the sidewalks or even the gutters in front of their homes. On cold winter days, they wore heavy coats.

It was a source of unspoken pride to have a clean sidewalk and gutter. Otherwise, guests might be offended when they came to call.

Brisk strokes — right, left, right — provided a good workout in the morning.

One's front porch also had to be swept daily to clear away leaves, dust, or even accumulated snow that had blown in overnight. A clean entry meant a good housekeeper lived there.

Nana had never been rich. My grandfather was a coal miner with a fourth grade education. He never earned much money, but Nana's philosophy was, "Soap, water, and elbow grease don't cost much."

She had also had her own share of medical problems, having been diagnosed with uterine cancer when she was 40 and having had several heart attacks over the years. But she never exhibited a victim mentality.

Whenever Nana got angry with my grandfather, instead of exchanging harsh words, she'd grab her broom and stomp outside to take out her frustrations on the sidewalk, sometimes almost refinishing the cement with her swift, hard strokes. When she came back inside, her anger seemed to have been swept away as well.

If she became lonely after my grandfather died, she could be seen softly sweeping leaves from the sidewalk, waiting for a passerby or neighbor to join her for a few words. She would chat, leaning on the broom, her ever-present companion. Nana taught me many things about how to live and cope. She also showed me that there is something almost sacred about having a clean porch, stairs, and sidewalks waiting to greet guests, no matter what kind of a house you live in.

Healing Words

When the class assignment is to focus on a family member and write about him or her, the class members do their normal thing. They take about 10 minutes to write, and then when I ask if anyone wants to read, a few hands go up. I never know what to expect when someone starts to read; neither do others in the room. Some family memories generate anger; others bring deep sorrow or regret. Others are just plain funny. As we go around the room and people read, some students cry and others laugh. I keep tissues handy for all occasions.

Mandy was my student when I taught high school. Over the years, as she rose through the ranks of television news producers, she returned to my college journalism classes as a guest speaker. We always kept in touch even as she took jobs at television stations around the country, got married and had a daughter, and moved to France. It was only recently, when she wrote to tell me that her mother had died of cancer, that I asked her if she wanted to join Writing for Wellness as an email student. She agreed and has completed several writing assignments. Here is the latest.

Tell Me about Your Mom

My therapist asked me to tell her about Mom. I paused, looked up to the ceiling to gather my thoughts, and jumped in. The first thing that popped into my mind: Mom loved to laugh. And she knew everything. She could beat the pants off anyone in Trivial Pursuit and took great pleasure in doing so (without gloating, mind you). She loved to read and watch movies and television shows about history or mysteries.

Nothing was more important to her in the world than her family. She was an only child, but felt that her cousins were the sisters she didn't have. She loved animals — two huge dogs and a tiny cat. Mom always had a story about what one or all of them had done.

Mom enjoyed traveling and museums. Travel didn't have to mean packing a bag to go around the world. But Mom took me to England and Scotland for my college graduation gift. I'll never forget the day we sat people watching in a park in Edinburgh. Years later, she and I would talk about the woman with her Springer spaniel sitting alongside her on the park bench. And we couldn't talk about our trip without talking about the woman in the pump room in Bath — the one who set off her camera flash in her own eyes. Or the two "brothers" from South Carolina we met on the train to Scotland — and their warning to us that Yorkshire pudding wasn't a dessert.

When my daughter Kaitlyn was born, Mom stayed with us for a couple of weeks. Every night for those weeks, she slept holding Kaitlyn on her chest. "The human mattress" she called herself. When Kaitlyn needed to eat, Mom would wake me up and I'd stumble out to the couch where we discovered just how bad TV programming is at 3 a.m., even with cable. We'd laugh at HGTV's Weekend Warriors and their complete inability to handle the project they'd taken on — or turn up our noses in disgust at the creations churned out in the kitchen stadium.

But whatever it was we watched, we laughed. And she made those feedings not so bad. She also taught me that it doesn't matter what you sing to a baby. They just like music. So she sang the IU fight song, over and over, and made me feel better about not knowing the words to much more than the Brady Bunch.

Mom was also fiercely loyal — not just to her family but also to her friends and to her employees — anyone who'd earned it.

She stood behind my brother Patrick and me in whatever we wanted to do, even when no one else did, even when it seemed crazy. Her phone line was open 24/7. And I took advantage of it.

Mom never judged or scolded. Sure, she corrected and advised. But it was always, always from her heart.

Today was the first time I'd even thought about Mom the way she was before she was diagnosed with cancer. It made me smile. It made me feel good. It felt really good to know that someone so wonderful had been such a big part of my life. It was good to know that someone so wonderful had taught me so much. And it was good to know that I can keep all that alive in my heart. Thanks Mom. For everything.

— **Mandy Murphy-Radeline**

Theda said she always thought of herself as a problem solver. But, when her 37-year-old daughter's cancer returned, that was one problem she realized, as a mother, she couldn't solve.

Oh, Mother! Please

This is a tortured-mind day in the life of the mother of a cancer patient. Whenever I get overly analytical or delve into suppositions, Donna always gives me this, "Oh mother! Please!" bit. Figure out how to make lemonade from these lemons. Anger is one way to deal with pain, but you have to be very careful not to let it spill over into the space of the people you love. Where's God, damn it? I can't find God. I pray; it's empty.

I figure He already has His mind made up and what right do I have to ask for anything? I haven't been the Christian person that I was in my youth. Going to church is a big pain in the neck. I'd much rather be gardening on my God-forsaken hillside on Sunday morning.

I think I'm still a believer, but I have to admit it's bloody murky in my old age. I think Christian people are much happier by far, but I can hardly stand the born-again zeal, and yet...

I just spent three days at Donna's home. Between her and her husband's work, the three girls, and sports schedules, tensions in the house run high. Everyone is constantly on the go.

It's very probably not as bad as I think it is right now. But as I see

Donna battling cancer, I am stressed with the pain of not being able to fix it.

— Theda Clark

When Christine reads anything she has written in class, there is always a moment of total silence as she finishes. People are spellbound. Her words are never routine, and the pictures she paints with them take all of us out of our own worlds. One class assignment I often give is to write about a person who is missing. When Christine finished her writing and raised her hand, I looked at her face and got the tissues ready, for her and for everyone in the room. Her title was her brother's name. We had all heard the name Francis Rex before.

Francis Rex

I look forward to the reunion with my brother, Francis Rex, one day. I know that it won't be for a while yet, but I know on that day, I will rejoice.

We will embrace again and be united. We will talk about the amazing life I was able to live and how he was there every step of the way.

We will recall our childhood memories and laugh and sing songs we remember.

We will bask in the glorious sun-love of heaven and give thanks for the time we had on earth.

He will show me all the work he has been doing, always so busy and yet always keeping watch over me.

I'll make some joke saying, "You've been such an angel," and then he'll gently remind me, "Don't forget you're one, too, now."

We'll peer down on our loved ones together and send blessings to earth...

I'll ask him, "Remember that day when I thought you sent me that sign? Was that really you?"

And he'll reply, "Well, I could have appeared as a ghost, but you told me you were afraid of ghosts so I had to resort to serendipity."

We will spend another eternity together, helping the world evolve into love. And then, we'll look at each other and say, "Hey, wanna give life another go? I'll see you when you get there."

— Christine Pechera

(Francis Rex Pechera died of cancer at age 16 following a failed bone marrow transplant. Christine was his donor.)

To follow such a poignant piece was too much for some members of the class who previously had wanted to read their writings. They simply put down their hands. "Too hard to follow that," someone says.

"Well, anybody got anything lighter?" I ask.

Edna is already smiling as her hand goes up.

Breakfast of Champions

No one ever said that getting through school was easy. But who would have thought that first grade would be rife with moral and ethical traumas?

Well, it happened to me.

Here I am, six years old, a "good girl," used to obeying parents and any other authority figure, for that matter.

I can still see the classroom: small tables and smaller chairs where we do our work of reading and writing. There is also the area for story time and show and tell.

Our teacher, Miss Chambers, sits in her upright wood and metal chair, while we kids sit at her feet, cross-legged on the oblong braided area rug, looking up in rapt attention for whatever words of wisdom will come from our respected teacher-god.

First thing every morning, we little students plop down on that rug and wait for Miss Chambers to speak.

This morning, seemingly out of the blue, Miss Chambers announces, "Let's go all around the room and find out what we ate for breakfast."

Now that should not be difficult. One by one, Susan and Jeffrey and Billy list what they ate for breakfast: toast and jam, oatmeal, corn flakes, Wheaties, orange juice, milk, etc.

Now it is my turn. "I ate a roll with cream cheese and coffee," I announce proudly.

Miss Chambers' face turns a strange shade of pasty white and her mouth freezes, "You had what for breakfast?" she asks.

I repeat my morning repast.

Her eyes narrow and she says to me in a stern voice, "You cannot drink coffee and have that breakfast. You must have cereal and milk and orange juice. You tell your mother to start giving that to you for breakfast. I'll ask you again tomorrow and I expect you to eat properly!"

Blood rushes to my face as I feel the humiliation and shame flood throughout my body. Here I am wanting to do only good, and now Miss Chambers is angry at me AND my mother. This is trouble, big trouble.

All that day I think about how I can solve my problem without upsetting anyone.

My six-year-old brain finally hits on this: I will simply talk to my mother, tell her what Miss Chambers said, and ask her to give me cereal, milk, and juice for breakfast. "That will do it," I think to myself, feeling relieved.

Well, it does do it, but not in the way I hoped.

My mother is a grown-up good girl and she has always respected my teachers and the school administration.

But that afternoon when I go home and say, "Mommy, Miss

Chambers says you are not giving me a good breakfast. She wants you to give me cereal, juice, and milk for breakfast tomorrow," my mother's face immediately shows her surprise and anger.

"I don't care what Miss Chambers wants, I'm feeding you what I want. Tomorrow you just tell Miss Chambers you ate cereal for breakfast, that's all," she says, obviously still very annoyed.

Uh oh. Not the answer I want to hear. Now I am torn between my teacher-god and my mommy-god, who is also my food and shelter source. My stomach hurts real bad.

What am I supposed to do? The next morning, enjoying my roll, cream cheese, and coffee, I am scared but I have decided to lie to Miss Chambers.

When I walk through the school gate that morning, I feel as if I am going to my execution.

Miss Chambers will discover I am lying and will send me to the principal's office. I am doomed.

Sitting on the braided carpet, I wait as the other kids recite their breakfast menus, unaware that a liar is lurking in their midst.

Finally, it is my turn.

"And what did you have for breakfast this morning, Edna?" Miss Chambers asks expectantly.

Without hesitation, I reply in a strong voice, "I had cereal with milk, and juice."

I wait for lightning to strike me dead.

"Excellent!" Miss Chambers exclaims. "Now that's what I wanted to hear!"

"Exactly!" I think to myself.

I am better liar material than I have thought. Lightning doesn't strike, and I spend the rest of the day recovering from the emotional tug of war I have been through.

You may wonder if this incident started me on a crime wave of lying, cheating, stealing, and other socially unacceptable behavior. The answer is no. Future teachers rated me as a "good citizen" with "excellent work habits and cooperation."

I went on to lead a socially responsible life. Now sometimes I eat cereal, milk, and juice for dinner. But that's another story.

— Edna Teller

It's Your Turn

Do you have a Nana, a Rex, or another relative in your life that you want to write about? A profile of a person often includes what they looked and acted like and, most of all, what they said and did. As you write, try to paint a picture from memory of your family member. Introduce us and let us enjoy spending time with them.

Did you, as did Edna, experience a parent-teacher conflict? Or, have you, like Theda, been caught in the middle, wanting to "fix" the cancer for a loved one?

Give as many details as you can. Who said what to whom?

Jump Start

An example of one way to begin is below. Use the person's first name to begin.

... was always ... He/she always ... and loved to ...

Tell your story from that point, now that the reader has a picture of the person.

After you have finished your story, describe how going back in time and writing about it felt to you.

Chapter 25

Your Unspoken Dreams

Put on your wildest frock.
Dance merrily through the sky.
— Joy. E. Walker Steward

On New Year's Day following my first bout of cancer, my husband and I sat down to write a list of all the places we would like to see and all the things we wanted to do together before we died. It was a little uncomfortable uttering the D-word, but it did make the process meaningful and sobering. We weren't just blabbing or going through the motions.

Having cancer, like others who have also received that not-so-gentle tap on the shoulder reminding us all that life is not a dress rehearsal, has helped me realize how important it is to set goals.

Somehow, each of us knows how to write a "to-do" daily or weekly list of chores we want to accomplish. Check anyone's desk or kitchen table and you will probably find list upon list for all phases of house, car, and even personal maintenance.

Some people are obsessive about their lists and get a big thrill out of checking off completed projects. Those check marks create a sense of accomplishment. Getting things done is important business. I have even heard of people who write lists after they have completed the task, just for the exhilaration of checking off items. Go figure.

But, with all of the lists we all make, we rarely itemize our dreams.

So, Bob and I spent an hour or two on our dream lists. We had three: his, mine, and ours. Included on my personal list and our together list were to teach college, write a novel, visit England, ride the mules down into the Grand Canyon, get my pilot's license, and see Paris from the top of the Eiffel Tower. Our together list had many travel destinations and financial goals. Some of those plans were pretty expensive; some seemed well within our reach. Others just took time — lots of it.

Changing careers might even be next to impossible, especially with the cancer thing hanging over my head.

Bob, a former Air Force pilot, listed dreams of owning a small airplane and flying all over the U.S., perhaps to Alaska, maybe even to Europe. He also listed teaching college, writing a futuristic novel, and owning his own business.

We just let our minds go even if our pocketbooks might not be able to follow.

But, before I could accomplish much of anything, I had to regain my physical strength.

I enrolled in water aerobics classes at the local YMCA and have managed to attend five days a week for more than 20 years, rain or shine.

And, except for the pilot's license, which I am convinced was divine intervention to save my life and everyone else's on the ground, I have achieved all of the other personal goals. Getting cancer a second time was not on my list, but that's another story.

Just as with your own chores, you have a better chance of accomplishing them if you think they are important enough to write them down.

When I ask students to list their dreams/goals, it becomes evident immediately that those goals change, sometimes on a daily basis.

The writing tone and content of those who have gone through various stages of cancer diagnosis, treatment, and recovery reflect where they are in the process.

Writing for Wellness at any given time has a patient waiting for test results, another in pre-operative preparation, others counting down the hours for bone marrow or stem cell transplants, as well as some people who are in remission or have recovered completely.

The cancer-free survivors in class often serve as role models and inspirations to open the others' minds to the dreams they may have thought were lost.

My lesson on unspoken dreams is designed for the student to formulate plans and realize goals. As one class member put it, "I used up so much energy just surviving that I need to make a brand new life plan. I don't know who I am anymore or where I'm going."

Without a map, or at least a general idea of where you are heading, how could you know your destination?

Healing Words

Christine, then on the healthy side of her first bone marrow transplant, gained renewed strength and insights each day. What started with fear and anger transitioned into a new perspective, one she was determined to retain for the rest of her life. Her guidelines provided life direction to everyone.

January 25

Let go of the "couldas" and the "shouldas." Your life has unfolded exactly as it should have, and the "couldas" are in the past and the past does not exist in the now.

The past limits your mind to the linear constraints of time. The universe is now. Trust in it.

Use your will and recognize opportunity. Use love and be righteous. But do not hang all your thoughts on outcome.

Life is living. It is catching that wave, hitting that target, dancing to the rhythm, allowing that kiss to flow completely through you. It is not to be the fastest, the most powerful, most wealthy, or most popular. These may be side effects of your efforts to live fully, but they should not be your goals. Life is a quest and that quest is for one singular moment, a complete and timeless moment, when all at once you feel joy, elation, relief, and oneness. When you are in rhythm with the symphonic pulse of the universe, you can feel the electrifying current of the life force, a hundred thousand gigawatts of light bursting out of each and every cell.

When fear completely dissolves into non-existence, at that moment, the whole busy world fades away and it is just you and that ocean, that mountain, that face. And nothing could be more right. There are no questions, no doubts. The unknown is welcomed with relish. That is heaven.

— Christine Pechera

Anna was in the midst of treatments for colon cancer when she joined Writing for Wellness class. Her dream is to get well and return to the Kern River, one of California's most beautiful mountain waterways.

Kern River

Flow to me softly from the mountains on high,
   where the trees try to reach toward the clear blue sky.
Rush though the valleys where the animals graze,
   flow through the meadows with the flowers ablaze,
Flow to me softly for I'll be there someday
   to touch your clear waters as you pass my way.

— Anna Andrizzi Escobosa

Linda has worked in Patient Services for City of Hope for nine years. After her recovery, she followed her unspoken dream. Ironically, what started as a very personal goal ended up helping fellow breast cancer sisters in a once-in-a-lifetime experience. She had come full circle.

I Did

I was 16 years old. My boyfriend had one. I loved it. My mother would have killed me if she ever knew. When I was 21, my ex-husband got one. I was totally hooked.

That was more than 25 years ago, but I never forgot — the sound, the look, the thrill, the coolness.

But I was a girl, for heaven's sake. We didn't do that sort of thing! Did we?

It nagged at me, it intrigued me, and it made me smile. I filed it away somewhere in the back of my mind — for later.

After my 1996 cancer diagnosis, things changed. I began to think about my "life list" — things I'd always wanted to do, but had put off for one reason or another.

No longer.

I quit an unfulfilling job, volunteered, took up watercolor painting, went back to college, and took two trips to Maui. I got a dog, got rid of one annoying parrot, and bought a BMW.

But, there was still that one, unfinished thing.

My husband of more than 18 years, who previously had no interest whatsoever in them (until a couple of friends got theirs) actually started the process.

He bought them for my 47th birthday — the lessons, that is.

We went to the local community college and took the 19-hour course.

We passed.

We went to the Department of Motor Vehicles and took the test.

We passed.

A friend was selling his and we bought it. For me.

After a lifelong fantasy, my black and chromed 2003 Dyna Super Glide motorcycle proudly shared our garage. My husband got his shortly after mine.

Although I started practicing in the school parking lot, I went around the block a few times by myself. After all, it took me a little time to get comfortable on something that weighed 622 pounds!

And yes, unfortunately, I dropped it on its side once. Fortunately, it didn't even sustain a scratch, only a broken front brake lever along with my pride.

And yes, my mother would still kill me if she found out.

As a good friend reminded me, "Life's too short; get a Harley!"

I did.

— Linda Baginski

(Changing Gears, a group of young breast cancer survivors, with Linda's help, raised more than $60,000 for breast cancer research by riding their Harley motorcycles from San Diego to San Francisco and then again taking part in a ride across Australia in 2005.)

It's Your Turn

Anyone can do this. It doesn't take a "writer" to begin. No "Jump Starts" are required. Make a list of your personal goals. One category might be physical/health goals. Another might be family or career goals. A dream of global peace and understanding might be your choice for a topic. Traveling might be another category.

Next select one of the goals. Write about how it would feel to accomplish it. Someone once said, "If you can dream it, you can do it." Assume that is correct.

Here are some instructions on writing about how you can dream up a dream trip:

Where would you like to travel? Who would you take with you? Let your mind wander and try to picture yourself having a great time in a place you have always wanted to visit, a place where you will feel wonderful.

Concentrate on what the place will look and sound like. What would it smell like there? How will the foods taste? Use your five senses to bring out the complete picture. This dream trip is very cheap; it will only cost you some ink and paper.

Take a dream trip when pain, stress, or people drag you down.

After you are finished writing, check your list and ask yourself what steps will you need to take to accomplish a goal you selected? One radio psychologist suggests we take a 3x5 card and write some of our goals on the card, carrying it with us in our wallet or purse.

When we are faced with choices on how to spend time or money, we should take out the card and ask, "It this going where I want to go?" If not, choose to spend your time, money, or energy for something that is.

Chapter 26

Rediscovering You

My world is wide open. I have choices.
My life is a great blank slate.

— Christine Pechera

Having cancer or experiencing a life-changing tragedy provides a time for reflection, time that the "untouched" may not fully understand.

I got out of bed one night about midnight and without turning on the lights, I walked around our house, looking out at the lights of Los Angeles sparkling below our foothill home. My thoughts were strange. I had just been diagnosed with cancer.

I wondered how long I would live, but for the first time, I realized — completely — that it would not be forever. On a logical level, I had always known that. Everybody knows that.

But that night it became as crystal clear as those city lights. It was not a frightening experience, but it was not pleasant either, more of a combination. I realized that my life was finite. Thoughts of heaven or the afterlife were not there. I was thinking only of life on earth, life with my husband, life with my family, life in that house, that city, that earth. Just reliving it now brings tears to my eyes.

It wasn't long after that, though, that I felt a sense of urgency to spend wisely whatever time I had left. To waste time would be, just that, a waste. Feeling sorry for myself was also a waste of time. It would change nothing.

I made a pact with myself to make each day count. That didn't mean I cleaned closets, organized the garage, or even made specific career plans. I realized that those activities would somehow get done — or not.

For me, making each day count sometimes means just walking in a park and celebrating life. Other times it means reading a good book from start to finish, becoming totally absorbed and thrilled by the process.

Following my first bout with cancer, I heard radio psychologists in Los Angeles talking about people's "life scripts." If your life was depressing and a mess, it was, they seemed to be saying, your own fault.

I remember one of them said something like, "Decide who you are and how you are going to live your life — just like you would write a script for a play or a movie. Then ask yourself if the movie script for your life is going to be a comedy, a tragedy, a drama, or one of those artistic movies no one can explain when the credits roll."

As simplistic as that concept sounded, I felt it was very good advice.

The psychologist went on to tell listeners to decide who was going to play major acting roles in their script and who would be "cut" from the cast. That, too, was an interesting concept. Many times I wondered why I had involved myself with overly negative people who I seemed to be carrying around without getting any personal satisfaction from. I also didn't seem to be helping them. Trying to cheer someone up who refuses your help seemed futile. Losing causes I didn't need. Apologies to Mother Theresa.

The final bit of pop psychology advice about choosing the ending of your life's script intrigued me.

I wrote my script, chose a small cast of meaningful players, selected a story with feeling and impact on others, and made a conscious decision to have a happy ending. I also wanted it to be a simple story, one that everyone could understand. Then, it was time to live it and rediscover life and myself in the process.

The line from the old Johnny Mercer tune, "Accentuate the positive, eliminate the negative, latch on to the affirmative, and don't mess with Mister In-Between," has become the background music.

Healing Words

When I ask students to write about their new lives, they all seem to understand what I mean. I tell them about the idea of the life script, but I don't have to elaborate much. They get it.

I give them several choices for writing topics. One is to think about all of the goals they have in their lives. Then they are to select the ones that, following their battle for survival, they would still like to keep on their lists. Their lists are short; their goals are direct and have to do with quality of life, not quantity of material goods — somewhat predictable. Somehow, though, the act of writing lists makes them seem more real.

Another topic is that of the crossroads. I ask them to write about any choices they might have been facing and to examine the pros and cons of each choice. Again, the choices they write about almost always relate to quality of life/health and their hopes for fulfilling relationships.

Personal advancement through education or training is also important to many students, especially the ones in the 20 to 50 age range. Going back to school to take art, music, and writing courses seems to resonate with every group of survivors.

The first step for all of them, it seems, is to fully recognize that a new perspective exists. Their writings reflect their changed lives.

Christine had just recovered from the first transplant when she addressed other survivors from her new perspective, one she achieved in her own passage to recovery. But soon after writing this, despite her hopes, she found herself a patient again.

Patient No More

It will come differently for different people. The day when you can take down the "Get Well" cards. When the numbers of your doctors and hospitals can come off the refrigerator. When you don't need to keep your medications next to your bed anymore. There will be a day when you can put all these things away, perhaps even throw them away.

That's when you recognize, honor, and then let go of your identity as "patient" and embrace the new you, your new body and self that you have evolved into. This day cannot be forced. Its arrival cannot be speeded up. It cannot be staged. Yet one day, you will arrive home. You will wake up and you will realize that the many medical things around the house no longer pertain to you. You will know. When that day comes, make it a quiet, graceful embrace. Be silent and pray for the many who did not make it this far. Give thanks for the love and support you received during your trial/challenge/fight/opportunity.

Thank your illness for the lessons it taught you. Then say goodbye to it. Step out.

Imagine that you have been in a fenced yard during this experience. Now the gate is open and you step out, out of the yard, outside the fence. You are free. Feel the sun on your face, the breeze on your cheeks, the fresh delicate air nourishing your nose and filling your lungs with delight. Look ahead. What do you see?

Step forward. It's all yours.

— Christine Pechera

After Janet's cancer treatment failed, she needed a stem cell transplant. Following its success, she emerged with renewed faith.

A Blessing

God blessed me just the other day,
Gave me a second chance on life, showed me the way.
God in his glory, angels beaming from above,
Waiting for me to start my new life with all of their love.

— Janet Gray

Bill's thanks his bone marrow donor for anonymously giving him the chance to rediscover life and himself.

Letter to My Bone Marrow Donor

What do you tell someone who every day is giving you the gift of life — someone you do not know, someone who might be anywhere around the globe?

In today's world, where the selfishness and egos of a few take center stage, the compassion, caring, and faith of people like you go largely unpublicized. Yet, with my sickness, I've come to realize that those, such as you, do not seek open reward or publicity for your gift. Your reward is inward, spiritual in whatever personal or organized faith you practice.

While I always believed in the inherent goodness of people everywhere, my current health challenge verified that faith, and has made me aware of just how many compassionate and caring people there are. Your gift of life has given me a new birth; I have a future and can continue to look forward to things I love including:

Being with my wife, working in the garden, watching things grow.

Seeing my children mature, and my grandchildren grow up.

Getting a travel trailer and going camping and fishing.

Returning to Europe.

Finally attending a Rolling Stones concert and a "Homecoming" football game.

Finishing the western novel I started writing.

Cooking and enjoying a meal with a nice glass of wine — maybe even wine I made. I simply cannot convey what that means to me.

Having a future is too special. For putting the needs of a stranger first, bless you for your gift.

— **Bill Matteson**

It's Your Turn

Who have you become? Have you rediscovered new parts of your personality? Have hidden aspects of your being suddenly re-emerged? Write a brief "life script" describing the life you hope to live from here on. Who will be in the cast? Were some people around you told, "Don't call us; we'll call you." Will it be a drama, a comedy, or an inspirational story? Does it have a happy ending? Or, if this is too big of an undertaking right now, you may simply want to write about what you will do with your new freedom.

Jump Start

Since I am the "author" of my life script, I want life from here on to be ...

Cancer (or a tragedy) has given me a new outlook. I have become a new person ...

Once you get started, your own thoughts and words will take over.

Chapter 27

Giving Back

What will you do with the love you have to give?
It is useless to keep it to yourself.
— Christine Pechera

When my husband was asked to run for our local city council, he was dumbfounded. Margaret Finlay, our neighbor, the mayor, approached us as we packed our car for a vacation. She told Bob that a group of 25 people had signed a petition nominating him. Huh? He was a full-time university professor teaching aerospace engineering.

They were begging him to run, Margaret said. "You're smart; you're honest! We need you!"

He protested loudly, "But, I'm not a politician!"

"That's exactly why we want you!"

I remember reading once that the best leader is often a reluctant one — no hidden agendas. He fit that bill. He reluctantly agreed to run for our local city council. He campaigned, won by a landslide, and served four years, giving back to our community and serving his final year in office as the mayor. The townspeople still want him to run again.

He still protests, "I'm not a politician."

But, when asked what the best part of serving was, he often says, "Meeting all the wonderful people who volunteer throughout the city, the ones who really make everything happen."

I loved seeing my husband make a difference. But, as his wife, I didn't appreciate people who protested a decision they disliked and interrupted council meetings with the nasty comments such as, "All politicians are crooks!" or snarled, "You can't trust any of them!"

Bob, more understanding than me, agreed with Harry Truman's comment, "If you can't stand the heat, stay out of the kitchen." And Bob, like Harry, stayed in the kitchen.

Prior to his political involvement, when I watched the national elections, I always wondered who would ever want to subject themselves to the open scorn of protestors.

But, thankfully, in our town as in most towns, there is a group of wonderful and positive volunteers who make the time spent in the public arena a very positive one. It is they who, quietly and without asking for any recognition, make everything happen for the schools, the seniors, the needy, and, most importantly, the good of the entire city. We always see the same faces at all of the fund raising events for charities, the library board, the historical society, the Chamber of Commerce functions, drug-prevention committees, soccer and youth baseball, the women's club, Rotary, Lions, Elks, you name it.

If there is a scholarship to be given to a worthy high school student, one of the faithful will be standing outside in the rain in front of our local supermarket with a donation jar. If the Brownies or Girl Scouts are selling cookies or the Boy Scouts are asking for help to get to camp, there are those same people keeping the kids company and being sure they are polite and making correct change.

Serving one's community has its own special rewards and, as one stalwart volunteer once explained, "Doing good feels good!"

My five-plus years (and counting) as the volunteer teacher of Writing for Wellness classes have given me untold happiness and fulfillment. I feel I belong right there in that funny little room — that wildly decorated comedy theatre where Bart Simpson stares back at me from one wall and Garfield the cat grins from another. The moments my students and I have shared — the highs and the lows — are all steps toward our collective healing.

Giving back is getting.

Healing Words

During the most traumatic phase of cancer treatment, no patient is able to give back to anyone. It is impossible. Relying on everyone else is simply the name of the game. Then, gradually, as pain and fear subside and energy creeps back, thoughts of helping pull others through their dark days start to play with the healing mind. Soon those thoughts germinate into ideas and ideas bloom into plans.

Recently named our town's first poet laureate, Robert Prado now writes uplifting poems for all major city events. Robert's other way of "giving back" sometimes takes place in the hospital parking lot.

Ships

On my way to the hospital where I go now and then for checkups and medicine, I passed a frail looking man walking slowly across the parking lot. I touched him on the shoulder and he turned around.

Pain was written all over his face. I said to him, "I was like you three and a half years ago."

He told me he had lung cancer, but after his surgery and chemo, his last report said he had "stabilized."

"I know you'll have a lot of bad days and a few good ones, but later on your days will be reversed," I told him. "You're like a little, frail weed that with hope and determination breaks through the asphalt."

He replied, "Thanks. You've given me hope."

We shook hands and, as I turned to leave, I felt like I was on one ship and he was on another, passing opposite each other — too far apart to touch, but somehow we did.

— **Robert Prado**

Dori, at the height of her career and the CEO of her own company, was also taking advanced courses at the local university when she learned she had melanoma. She is a continuing patient at City of Hope and chooses to give back to those who find themselves alone and fearful as they face the same disease.

Surviving by Giving Back

The diagnosis was melanoma, the most advanced kind of skin cancer. I felt heartbroken and angry at the same time. But I found out about my cancer through another person who was "giving back" by publicizing the disease.

One evening I had been watching one of those talk shows when the late Maureen Reagan was being interviewed. I did not know a lot about Maureen at that time and I was interested in what she had to say as she openly discussed her battle with melanoma. She stressed the importance of seeing a dermatologist for a skin check up. I called my dermatologist the next day.

Then my life changed.

In a series of events that took me from specialist to specialist and the diagnosis from basal cell cancer to malignant melanoma, my emotions were on a roller coaster. What would happen to me? What if I didn't make it through? Where could I find other melanoma patients to talk to?

After surgery, I was told by my doctors that the melanoma had been caught in an early stage. I would survive. Two more major surgeries followed within a year. But are our battles ever really over? I have a new small tumor on my right lung that my doctors are tracking.

In the meantime, I decided to give back to the place and the people who cared for me, the people I trusted the most and those I considered to be my "family."

After going through special training, I am one of the designated people who patients can talk to when they are first diagnosed.

I also address groups on sun safety and ways to prevent skin cancers. Like lung cancer, melanoma is preventable. Raising awareness about this disease is my way of giving back. If I can help save one life, then I have given back tenfold.

Lee Ann Womack's song, "I Hope You Dance" is an inspiration to me.

I am dancing now and I know that this continuous journey means sharing and helping others. Giving back is the best part of life and I hope others will learn to take this challenge as well.

— Dori Ann Neuman

Joan told about how she learned to give back after getting cancer.

A Rekindled Light

As a high school student and later on in college, I always thought of myself as a doer. I was on the newspaper and was business manager of the yearbook. In college, I was on both the newspaper and humor magazine, in addition to editing the dorm newsletter. There were always things to do — fun things that gave me a sense of accomplishment and created a circle of friends.

Marriage, children, and moves across the country put an end to that. Without realizing it, my optimistic view of life became a pragmatic one. I was still "doing," but doing what had to be done rather than what I enjoyed. My friends narrowed to only a few close ones, partly because of distance but primarily because the efforts required seemed too much for me. There were so many other things that "had" to be done. In addition, there were two bouts of depression to add to the mix.

Five years ago, cancer, that scary, sometimes painful, and always debilitating disease, made me stop, look around, and realize what I'd been missing. I knew it was time for a change. Since I had always loved being around children, and even my grandchildren were rapidly growing up, I decided to volunteer for the Grandparent Reading program at my library. I now read to an elementary school class on Literacy Day and mentor a third grader who needs some extra attention. There is nothing like being around a child to let you know what is really important and that fun is an important element of life.

I joined Writing for Wellness class, its members now counted among my dearest friends. Although I live more than 40 miles away, distance never deters me from being with my friends.

I have become a volunteer for the American Cancer Society's Reach for Recovery Program, and through that group have met many soul sisters. I have also become a mentor for a teenaged mother, and hope that our relationship makes clear the need for love and laughter in everyone's life.

Every day, I try to make time for a walk by the ocean, a view of the sunset, and a chance to touch base with at least one person in my once-again widening circle of friends. Once more, I've become a doer with a zest for life, a smile for everyone, and just a bit of attitude.

Albert Schweitzer said, "Sometimes our light goes out but is blown into flame by another human being. Each of us owes deepest thanks to those who have rekindled this light." Thanks to all who have rekindled mine.

— Joan Smith

Janet tells her story and explains how and why she is giving back.

My Story

Being a volunteer at the City of Hope has turned out to be the best job I have ever had. My title is "Patient Escort." I escort cancer patients to meet their new doctors. All patients are different; some choose to walk down the hallways in silence; others would rather talk about what is going to happen to them. I can see the fear in their eyes, the same fear I had when a volunteer escorted me and my husband to my first doctor visit. I remember being frightened about the uncertainty ahead.

Patients I escort now ask me, "Why are you a volunteer?"

I answer, "I am still a patient here, but my disease has been in remission for eight years now."

They look at me in astonishment and tell me they are facing a stem cell or bone marrow transplant. I explain that I had a stem cell transplant eight years ago. The looks on the patients' faces are priceless.

Everyone's situation is certainly different, but when patients see someone like me, someone who has been through it and is still standing here and enjoying life, it gives them hope, too.

It shows them a little light at the end of the tunnel and tells them that all things are possible. I go home at the end of the day with a very warm heart and a contented feeling, knowing I have truly tried to help someone. Isn't that what life is all about?

— Janet Gray

Annie was one of 9,000 participants in the annual Walk for Hope to raise money for breast cancer research and to honor survivors as well as those whose lives were taken by the disease. It is a 5K and while many participants are elderly, some are younger but out of shape, and lots of others are under-prepared for the workout. But, as they endure the physical trial and repeatedly put one foot in front of the other, participants come away from the experience realizing it is not about them. It is about the women who they represent and what their lives mean to each person walking. Annie's soft and lyrical voice made listeners in class feel as if we, too, were walking and walking in rhythm.

Walk for Hope

It's for my sister, my best friend,
The whole time we were growing up,
She was always there for me.
So now I'm walking and walking.
Never forget, never forget.

It's for my sister, too.
We never were close, until the end.

But, thank God, I could be there for her.
So now I'm walking and walking.
Never forget, never forget.

It's for my Mom
She's had cancer three times now.
I don't want to lose her.
So I'm walking and walking.
Never forget, never forget.

It's for my baby girl,
Such a beautiful young woman.
It's not right for a man to bury his child,
So I'm walking and walking.
Never forget, never forget.

It's for my Grandma,
She made me cookies and made me laugh,
I miss her stories and her warm smile,
So I'm walking and walking.
Never forget, never forget.

It's for my wife,
The love of my life,
Mother of our three sons,
So I'm walking and walking.
Never forget, never forget.

It's for my wife, too,
Fifty years together just isn't enough,
I cry myself to sleep every night,

So I'm walking and walking.
Never forget, never forget.

It's for my patients,
That I care for each day,
Their courage and strength inspire me,
So I'm walking and walking.
Never forget, never forget.

I have a wife, a sister,
A daughter, a mom,
Dear God, I pray it doesn't
Happen to them.
I pray they find a cure.
So, I'm walking and walking and walking.

— Annie Watson

*The death of Lynn's father had a profound effect on her career path.
She chose to leave academics to join the battle against cancer.*

From Helpless to Hopeful

That October morning started off routinely enough. Up early and out
the door before the sun stretched its rays fully across the sky, I was at
my desk in the academic dean's office at the college when the first bell
rang starting the school day.

From my office window, the students looked like tired ants moving
towards the classroom building, shoulders stooped under the weight of
their books. Their glazed looks reminded me of my own days of too little
sleep and too much computer time.

By lunchtime, I was chatting with students who were happy to be finished with classes and looking forward to an afternoon of sleep, play, or work. As they disappeared into the sunshine, I turned to my desk, mentally reviewing the tasks ahead.

In the next moment, everything changed. My priorities suddenly became reordered. When is a good time to get a call that your dad has cancer?

The conversation unfolded as I expected it must for many people hearing the news for the first time from a distance.

"What did you say? Dad? What happened? When did he find out?" followed by the always, "Are they sure?"

Helplessness tightened its fingers around my throat making each question hard to ask.

I had never used the words dad and cancer in the same sentence. My knowledge of cancer was limited to the bout my mom had weathered when diagnosed with colon cancer several years before. She had undergone surgery and had been cancer free for years.

My dad's doctor explained that they had "caught the cancer on the adrenal glands," but that it was too far advanced for chemo.

The outlook was dismal, perhaps two months at the most. Upon hearing the news, the "flight or fight" response that comes when you feel threatened held true for me. I immediately arranged for my young daughter, Abby, and me to fly home to spend 10 days with Dad before the illness had time to overtake him.

My head hurt from the questions that wouldn't stop. Why him? Why now? What about us?

We understood so little. We only understood that we'd joined the growing numbers of those who sit with their loved ones in oncology waiting rooms. Waiting. Always waiting. We listened to others bare their hearts with abandon. "He never smoked, he never drank, he never said a bad word, and now they say he has throat cancer? How can this be?"

one distressed wife asked of no one in particular.

During the 10 days we were in Illinois, Abby and I spent as much time as we could with Dad and his adorable little mongrel, Shorty. Having never had a family pet, both of us grew attached to this little mop of a dog who stood barely one foot off the ground.

We also came to be in his debt as we realized that Shorty took the night vigil with dad as he sat up in his chair, willing himself to see another dawn.

Never one to take medication, Dad was taking an obligatory aspirin a day to combat the pain from the disease that was ravaging his body. It wasn't until several days into our trip that I realized why the sports channel played so loudly in the background 24 hours a day. The sound from the television masked Dad's moans.

Almost five years after my dad passed away, I gained a different perspective on cancer when I became part of the administrative staff at City of Hope. The helplessness I felt watching my dad slip away had abated somewhat as I earned my own place in the battle.

I have found an organization with outstanding research and patient care that is dedicated to finding answers to the tough questions cancer patients and their families face.

I continue to see each day as a new opportunity to help our patients. My office may be in the hinterland of administration, but my heart is with those on the front lines, fighting daily against the disease. I count myself fortunate to be among an army of physicians, nurses, clinical staff, administrators, staff, and volunteers who wage that battle daily for their patients.

— **Lynn Palmer**

Linda Bergman, a Hollywood producer and screenwriter whose words you have read earlier in this book, was dying. She had fought

advanced leukemia for four years and then took herself off chemo, telling her doctor she wanted to go home to die. Her doctor insisted that she submit to one last clinical trial. She refused. But her daughter, Sarah, and her son, Adam, both then teenagers, and her husband, Chuck, pleaded with her. They couldn't imagine life without her.

Finally, she reluctantly agreed to give life one last try. Four months later she was completely cured. Now she volunteers at City of Hope each week giving reassurance to those who are walking the walk she knows so well. Linda can be found serving at the Patient/Family Resource Desk where the always-fearful new cancer patients come for information and guidance. Despite having deadlines to meet, screenplays to edit, executives to "do lunch" with, nothing, absolutely nothing can keep Linda from being there for patients. Her own life script demands it.

Free At Last

I have reached my goal. I am no longer the victim, but am assisting those who've come behind me. I see it on the patients' faces when I get the opportunity to say, "Oh, you have leukemia? I HAD that, too."

I see the light in their eyes as they search mine for answers. No, we don't always have the same disease, but they know I speak their language.

They know I can be trusted.

They know I have faced the demons and lived to tell about it.

They know I am disease free and standing in the midst of the storm shining a light to them.

They know I love them because I am them.

— **Linda Bergman**

It's Your Turn

Think about how you have been helped by someone, someone like Linda who was giving back. Write about how a certain individual made you feel.

Have you helped others by volunteering your time? If you haven't been a volunteer, think about how you might contribute. Maybe there is even a Writing for Wellness class in your future. Visualize yourself helping others and write about how it might feel?

Jump Start

When I helped ..., I felt ...

If I could volunteer my time or money, it would be to help ... because ...

Writing something down makes it more important. Words can be your plan for action.

Part V

One Family's Cancer Saga

Chapter 28

Steve's Story

I had the energy of a slug.

— Steve Rom

If it were a Hollywood movie script, its logline for TV Guide would read: Against all odds, a young man battles cancer, medical incompetence, and despair. Will he succumb or survive?

And, once the film came out, movie critic Leonard Maltin would give it his top rating: FOUR STARS. "Terrifying! Dramatic! Awe-inspiring! A must-see."

Other movie critics might disagree with Maltin's perfect score, though, saying the story was "over the top" or its characters were not believable. Even the ending might be considered too good to be true.

But, since truth is stranger than fiction, to be believed Steve's story needs to be told by eyewitnesses, including the author:

FADE IN

(Opening scene. Cast: Steve; his mother, Paula; the author and her Writing for Wellness students. The author narrates the scene.)

The Unforgettable Steve Rom

My first glimpse of Steve was on a cold, windy, and rainy day as I prepared the food and the room for my noon Writing for Wellness class in the Hope Village Comedy Theatre.

My "classroom" adjoins the lobby of the Hope Village registration area where cancer patients and their families check into the family living facilities on the grounds. There are 40 cottages and six RV spaces to accommodate people from out of town, out of state, and even out of the country who come to City of Hope for treatment and need to stay near the hospital or its treatment centers.

Families pay a nominal fee, much less than local motels or RV parks charge. Some people stay a night; others may be there for months as testing, treatment, surgeries, and follow-ups take place.

Members of my class who have stayed on the grounds comment that without those facilities, they couldn't possibly have afforded to have treatment so far from their homes. Patients also report that having their families so close by as they went through treatments kept them from sinking into depression.

Hope Village is aptly named.

But, just as at regular hotels and motels, there are check-in and checkout times.

Despite the pouring rain, I overheard a conversation that led me to believe the young man in his 20s, Steve, and his mother, Paula, had wanted to check in, but they couldn't because the previous residents had not yet checked out. Paula was also told she had paperwork to fill out.

Paula's voice sounded frustrated and disappointed. It was clear the delay had not been in their plans.

Steve, shivering, looked pale, thin, and exhausted. He collapsed in a chair next to my open door.

Obviously they weren't going anywhere very fast.

I continued to move furniture and set up the serving area, half-listening to what was going on in the lobby. It was about 10 minutes before class was to begin and I knew some of my students would be arriving soon. Others who lived more than an hour away usually showed up early, allowing time for traffic delays. I needed to finish my setup.

Chicken soup was on the menu, just the thing for a nasty day. The crock-pot was steaming.

"How about coming in for some soup?" I said, approaching Steve.

Steve looked up at me with sad eyes and a weak smile, "No thanks!" he grumbled, holding his head in his hands as he sat hunched over in the chair. His jacket was wet and he looked miserable, having walked from the parking lot almost a block away.

I felt very sorry for him and my rescuing personality plus my over-talking condition shifted into high gear as I blabbed in one long sentence.

"Really, it would warm you up! Come on in. We're having a class in Writing for Wellness and it's free, and you wouldn't have to stay, and..."

He started to protest again, but by this time I had almost pulled him out of his chair and continued to talk non-stop. I took advantage of his weakened state and broke him down.

He came, he ate, and he stayed for class. What I couldn't have known that day, though, was the series of events that had led Steve to City of Hope.

(Scene change: Hospital, Los Angeles. Paula picks up the story's narration from there. Cast includes various medical staff members.)

Mother, Primary Caregiver

Steve had been diagnosed with acute lymphocytic leukemia (ALL), a type of cancer that normally occurs in children. But he was in his 20s.

That unforgettable day began a lengthy process to prepare him for a bone marrow transplant, his only sure chance of survival.

My job was clear: to be Steve's primary caregiver during the intense transplant process. Since I am an orthopedic nurse by profession, the transition from mother to caregiver proved seamless.

My only focus, then, was getting my son back on his feet with as few complications as possible.

I was confident that I was ready for the task, but never could have anticipated all the snags that would arise.

Steve had to be put into "remission," an important task assigned to the teaching hospital just after he was diagnosed.

There, in the oncology ward, the most difficult part of being a caregiver began in earnest. It was an experience I can only describe as an exercise in frustration. From day one, it appeared their main focus was statistics rather than individuals.

Steve clearly was just another stop along the hallway for the "team" of doctors assigned to him, which included a head oncologist, an internist, a resident, a hematologist, and a fellow oncologist.

A few times Steve was not in his room when his team made their early morning and late afternoon rounds. Perhaps he was in the bathroom, or down the hall in the patient library.

In those cases, the team would just move on to the next room and wouldn't come back until much later in the day, if at all. Then I was the only one to keep track of Steve's blood counts, as well as his medications and the amounts being used.

Many times I found myself in charge of pre-medicating Steve for his spinal taps (lumbar punctures) and radiation procedures, all parts of the plan to rid him of the diseased red blood cells that had taken over 60 percent of his blood.

To administer Steve's medications, a pic-line had been inserted into his arm. The pic-line, a commonly used apparatus for cancer patients that eliminates the need for constant needle pricks, provided the permanent line into his vein. Through it Steve could receive chemotherapy, have blood transfusions, and have his lab work done without painful reinjections.

After my three decades of experience as a nurse, however, I was keenly aware of the possibility of complications arising from a pic-line inserted into an arm or a leg.

One major complication could be deep venous thrombosis, or severe blood clots, which can be life threatening.

In addition, a major staph infection could occur, which could result in a two-to-three-month delay of the transplant while IV antibiotics were employed to cure the infection.

As it turned out, Steve did develop a blood clot in his arm. Shockingly, his six doctors, his team, did not diagnose it. I had to diagnose it, and then couldn't get any of the doctors to agree with me until I insisted on getting a special ultrasound scan to confirm my findings. That fiasco, unfortunately, turned out to be just the beginning.

Steve's chemotherapy over the last three days at the hospital had to be administered via injection because his platelets and fibrinogen level (which clot the blood in the entire body) were severely low. This was another major oversight by the doctors.

They should have realized from Steve's daily blood work that the extreme chemotherapy dosages they had been administering had severely lowered his levels. Therefore no further injections should have been given. His blood had lost its ability to clot. My son could have bled to death.

When the oncologist finally arrived in Steve's hospital room, I told him we would be terminating the last three days of chemotherapy, and then explained why. He said fine and walked out of the room. But a few minutes later a nurse showed up with a chemotherapy injection. I was sitting at the time and promptly stood up.

I told this nurse to the stay by the door and not to move any closer. I gave her two choices: stay there and I would call the head of the oncology department and explain the situation, or she could go back to the desk and call him personally and advise him about what had just transpired.

There is no doubt that she would have killed Steve instantly had she given him that shot.

There were plenty of other problems at that facility, all of which I confidently say resulted from the doctors' lack of personal care and attention. Whenever they met with Steve in his room, they immediately began going over the day's upcoming procedures and reciting his blood counts even before saying hello to him. Frankly, there was no excuse for that.

If there was a silver lining to all of this, it was that we knew we would be leaving that hospital for the City of Hope, a national leader in bone marrow transplants.

(Scene change: Hope Village Comedy Theatre, Duarte, California. Cast: same as in opening scene. Paula continues her narration.)

It Never Rains in Southern California

What began as a dark and dreary rainy day in late April soon turned into a shining ray of hope.

The rain quickly drove us indoors as we arrived at the City of Hope where Steve was to receive a bone marrow transplant. We had arranged to stay in the Hope Village, the City of Hope's on-site family housing facility, along with Steve's grandmother, Pearl Cook. There we all would await Steve's admittance to the transplant ward, the BMT.

This was a trying time for all of us, one that began when my son was diagnosed in Arizona four months earlier. Thankfully, we were too busy with our newfound responsibilities to be slowed down by negative thoughts.

On this rainy morning, I was told to fill out the paperwork needed to check into our room at the Hope Village. Pearl, for her role, had to keep her thoughts positive to set a good example.

As for Steve, he just had to "ride out the storm," he said, which is something I presume had nothing to do with the weather that day.

As I carefully filled out forms at the Hope Village's check-in office, Steve sat on a chair in the waiting room behind me. He was dripping wet from the rain and, judging from his stoic look, appeared to be drowning in his thoughts. A few minutes later, something would jar both of us out of our reveries.

At the end of the hallway we heard rumblings through an open door. It sounded as if chairs were being rearranged and boxes moved. Someone was obviously getting ready for something. We noticed from a quick glance through the door that the room was painted in bright colors and adorned with giant pictures of cartoon characters. It looked like a nursery school, quite frankly.

Just then, a woman came out of the room and approached us.

Her hair and clothes were wet, apparently having just come in from the rain herself. She introduced herself as Julie Davey, and said she was going to teach a class in the nearby room in about half an hour.

It was called "Writing for Wellness," she said, and she went on to explain that she teaches it regularly to fellow City of Hope patients. Mrs. Davey, we learned, was a cancer patient. As full of energy and smiles as she was, frankly we were a bit surprised with that news.

Mrs. Davey said she would like us to participate in the class. That's when we discovered another one of her qualities: her persuasion.

Steve, you see, can be a tough nut to crack. And it appeared he didn't want to participate in anything on that day. But Mrs. Davey, to her credit, was just the nutcracker my son needed at the time.

Steve, ironically, is a sportswriter by profession. He was three years into his career at the *Ann Arbor News* in Michigan when he became sick and returned to Los Angeles, his hometown, to stay with me. He told Julie he was already a writer.

"Oh, that's terrific!" she replied, hearing about my son's job. "You'll love this class."

From the look on Steve's face, he clearly didn't want to participate. But there was no way he could say no to Julie. Nor could I. By the way, I now refer to her as Julie, not Mrs. Davey, because even at that early point it seemed she was a friend more than anything else.

For the next hour and a half, Julie was an instructor to my son, as well as about 20 other City of Hope cancer patients and some of their caregivers.

During the class, Steve wrote a story about some of our distant family members. The assignment that day was to write about an early positive memory. Steve wrote about the many times we visited this particular family for dinner parties when he was a child.

They were happy, innocent times, ones that Steve apparently still carried with him, even into his late 20s.

Other patients wrote about their own fond memories. Though the stories were vastly different in their subjects, the point was the same: to take their minds off their present situations, to free their thoughts and get them active, if only in their imaginations.

Later, Steve and I reunited in our cottage in Hope Village. He quickly handed me a prize he had won for the story he wrote that day. It was a small trinket, which a couple of other students in the class had also received for their writings. Steve said he won it for me, but that he felt guilty. When I asked him why, he said, "I'm a professional writer!"

He went on to explain he hadn't thought it was fair to the others in the class that he participated in what turned out to be a writing contest.

Ask any of his classmates that day, however, and I'm sure they all would have disagreed with him. They were a team now, a writing team, not simply a group of nameless cancer patients participating in a contest.

Julie, who we learned was a professor of journalism at Fullerton College just down the freeway from the City of Hope, made all this happen. To her, writing obviously was a passion as much as it was her profession.

By urging Steve to participate in the class, Julie helped take his mind off of the grim thoughts he was having that first day at the Hope Village. Not only that, but she helped my son plug back into his life as a writer. That, it turned out, became his lifeline during his upcoming month-long stay for his transplant.

I knew this for sure one bleak afternoon when he was simply too sick to attend Julie's writing class. He had been attending the classes, but when he couldn't on that day, Julie sent over a get-well card to Steve's isolation room. It was signed by each of the students in that day's Writing for Wellness class, all of whom sent along touching personal notes and drawings.

Julie, bless her heart, made all this happen. She was not just another writing teacher. She was not just another patient. She was an angel, one of many we met during our stay at City of Hope.

(Scene change: Hope Village cottage where Paula continues her narration. New cast member, Dr. David Snyder)

Nurse Paula's Story Continues

Those first four days at the Hope Village were a seemingly endless, 24-hour chemotherapy marathon. The goal was to zap Steve's blood counts to zero in order to prepare his body for the new, healthy blood he was going to receive during the transfusion.

He had been told that a worldwide search for a bone marrow donor had resulted in a match. We were ecstatic.

His transplant was scheduled for approximately 10 days later.

At the City of Hope, I found myself not having to worry about any mistakes. Everything going on there appeared to be routine for the doctor and his staff. Having just one doctor, a personal connection, was simply impossible to get at the other hospital.

My son and I were lucky enough to have that connection with Dr. David Snyder, the assistant director of oncology at the City of Hope, and an expert on ALL.

On one of Dr. Snyder's first visits to our room, Steve had left to take a walk. When I told this to our new doctor, I began to have nightmarish visions of the previous hospital. But it turned out they were unfounded, as Dr. Snyder proceeded to do something the other doctors never thought of: he went looking for Steve.

Dr. Snyder found him in the library down the hall and proceeded to hold his briefing with him there.

Later, Steve told me how stunned he was to see Dr. Snyder peek his head in the library door. "I couldn't believe it. That would have never happened at the other place," Steve told me.

Dr. Snyder, upon returning to our room later, smiled and explained, "I knew he couldn't go far."

With everyone at City of Hope being so accomplished at what they do, from cleaning personnel and parking attendants on up, I felt confident in letting my guard down. My mother, Pearl Cook, wasn't as relaxed.

Always the perfectionist, and forever the advocate for Steve, she did whatever she could to make sure things were going okay.

After each daily cleaning of Steve's room, and sometimes before, Nana, as Steve and his two cousins called her, tipped the cleaning personnel.

Steve, discovering this, became angry at Nana.

"Don't do that," he told her. "It's their job!"

But Nana was relentless, thus ensuring that Steve had the cleanest room on the oncology ward.

(Steve repaid his grandmother's favor years later. In March 2006 in Palm Springs, California, Steve tipped the hospital cleaning crew as his grandmother lay clinging to life. While her fight for life has ended now, Steve is certain that Nana knows what he did.)

(Change of scene: Dr. Snyder's office. The two main actors in this story, Steve and Dr. Snyder, speak their first lines. Steve narrates.)

No More Tears

I used the same words I had said before, pleading to the doctor at the previous hospital. "Save my life!" I belted, tears already flowing. "Don't do it for me. Do it for my family and friends who are suffering more than I am."

For that, the doctor at the previous hospital had patted me on the back. He went on to use words like if, might, maybe, perhaps in almost every sentence he used. I was not left with much confidence that I would or could survive.

Then I met Dr. David Snyder. Everything changed.

Dr. Snyder talked to me, in his reserved yet confident voice, saying, "When we find a donor, we will go ahead with the transplant and you are going to get back on your feet."

Since I am a big sports fan, as is Dr. Snyder, we both knew that when a coach addresses his team before an important game, he wants to be as confident as possible. Dr. Snyder had a game plan. When he spoke to me that day, I listened to it, I bought into it, and we both went out to play the game.

The final buzzer hasn't gone off yet but our team is way ahead.

(Change of scene: Hope Village cottage. Paula, alone, narrates.)

Paula Prepares for the Playoffs

I recuperated for the upcoming 30-day stay in the City of Hope when Steve would receive his bone marrow transplant.

I could be confident, finally, that we indeed had a winning "team" working with us.

We knew he was in the best possible hands.

(Change of scene: Sculptured Fountain, symbol of City of Hope, outside its main entrance. Steve narrates)

Hope Rises

Anyone who has ever seen the logo for City of Hope or who has ever been on its grounds has seen the modernistic statue "Hope Rises," the mother and father together holding their small child high above their heads.

At first glance, "Hope Rises" appeared to me to be just a catch phrase intended to drum up promotion. In reality, however, it became so much more.

I became well aware of this while receiving treatment for my acute leukemia.

Though things were going well in my recovery, I was still light years away from where I was physically and mentally before I was diagnosed.

It was six months after being handed that lump of coal for my Christmas present. It was just about two months after my May 4th bone marrow transplant. First, my immune system had to be zapped during an arduous one-month stay in the hospital — I had the energy of a slug — to prepare me for my transplant. Then, in the middle of the night, word came in that a donor, anonymous and unrelated to me, had been found who matched me perfectly and the donor's bone marrow was being driven from Los Angeles International Airport, having been collected and flown in from Germany! When it arrived, I was infused and immediately began my fight back to life.

My biggest task as I recovered at home in Los Angeles was making the 40-minute drive each way to City of Hope three times a week to receive outpatient treatments.

I was so burned out from the tons and tons of medications given to me during the transplant that even the seemingly simple task of leaving my apartment and riding along the freeways as my mother drove, was an exercise in frustration.

As the late-morning summer sun beat down on my frail skin, I felt about as comfortable as I would have if I stuffed myself into a clothes dryer and turned it on full blast. Each time I arrived in Duarte, I was rung.

Walking very, very slowly and with the aid of my mother, I passed the sculptured fountain with its Hope Rises statue.

That unique image, I recalled, was also on the lapel pins I had seen all the nurses wear. "Hope Rises."

I should have recognized the entrance to the hospital with its ice-cream smoothie stand, it colorful lawn chairs, and its friendly greeters I passed by as wonderful and welcoming. I didn't. Instead, I adopted the attitude of a teenage brat.

I scowled at that statue and said, smugly, "Hope Rises!"

My mom looked at me in confusion.

I repeated the phrase, each time more and more sarcastically, as if it was some deliberate attempt by the hospital public relations department to poke fun at my struggling situation.

"Hope Rises!" I uttered as I shook my head steadily in disgust.

But then, almost like magic, something happened in the middle of my mild temper tantrum. It was as if something switched on inside of me and I finally saw the light. I finally got it. I understood what "Hope Rises" meant.

This change to positive thinking occurred as I entered the infusion area in the Brawerman Clinic, primed to provide them the usual dozen or so vials of my blood.

Normally, that would irritate the heck out of me, a result mostly of all the bustling going on around me, nurses scurrying about, the IV machines beeping, the phones ringing.

But for some reason, that day, all I could do was smile and say, "Hope Rises."

It actually works, I thought. I uttered it over and over again with a smile on my face for the first time in months.

As mom and I drove home, suddenly, the sun didn't seem so blazing. And the freeways weren't so bumpy. Heck, there were even better songs on the radio, awesome songs that nearly inspired me to buy the CDs when I got back to my normal routine.

That's when it sank in, just why City of Hope chose "Hope Rises" as their motto, and put it on their statue, their pins, their stationery.

Six months after my bone marrow transplant, which was made possible by a total stranger whose marrow matched mine, test after test after test showed that I had 100 percent healthy donor blood in me.

I didn't need to say "Hope Rises" anymore.

I felt fine, better than I ever had in my life, in fact. I could muster enough enthusiasm, energy, and hope all on my own whenever I wanted.

I have now forgotten what it was like not to have the energy to walk across the room or take a leisurely drive on a sunny day.

But I'll never forget the power of that saying.

(Change of scene: Flagstaff, Arizona. Steve is sitting at the sports desk of the local newspaper. A pile of clippings — all of his recent articles — in front of him. He narrates.)

The Train

Life goes by at an alarming rate of speed. Rarely, if ever, do we notice anything more than a blur flashing before our eyes.

Then cancer strikes.

In an instant, the fast train we all find ourselves on once we reach adulthood comes to a sudden and screeching halt.

Actually, the train keeps moving. That train is life, and it includes a link of cars as far as the eye can see, each representing different stages of our journey as human beings.

No matter which car we had clung to when we were suddenly thrown off, we were all assigned to the side of the track.

"What happened?" eventually we asked. "What's to become of me?"

What happens next, actually, is all up to you. Will you cry? Pout? Get angry? Frustrated?

It's certain we've all experienced these reactions in one form or another. If we're lucky, once we come to grips with our fate, we decide on an attitude we're going to have during our journey back to health.

Whatever attitude you choose, in the long run it's important to remember one thing: The fast train you rode on for so long is now gone.

Forever.

It will not return. Things will never be the same. As cancer survivors, we are invariably much different from what we were prior to becoming sick. That's no secret.

What's more of a mystery is how we can actually benefit from going through such a frightening ordeal. Specifically, what can we learn from it?

The first thing you discover is who's going to be on board your new train once it arrives at the station. In other words, who leapt off their own train to rush to your side once hearing news of your illness?

And who didn't?

Who didn't even call you when you were in the hospital?

And who did?

Were the people you thought were "rocks" in your life suddenly crumbling and breaking away?

This was the time you needed those people — friends, relatives, co-workers — the most.

But, were people you thought were just faces in a crowd — or even sworn enemies — now reaching out to you?

While finding the answers to those questions, remember another thing: don't get too busy focusing your eyes on your bygone train as it gets smaller and smaller in the distance.

Instead, look around. Your eyes will widen at how many people actually share the same seemingly lonely spot you now occupy. They may not be sick, but they're there.

They're the nurses coming into your hospital room to change your IV bag. They're the people delivering your meal at the crack of dawn. They're the man or woman taking your weight and blood pressure every four hours.

These may all seem like meaningless tasks, but actually they're anything but. Like the people themselves, their tasks are your lifeline.

These people are the new rocks in your life.

Joining them are all those folks visiting you each day: friends, family members, volunteers from the Red Cross offering needed advice. Also, the authors of the stacks get well cards you receive each day, as well as the people calling you nonstop, even though you may be too sick or tired to accept their calls.

These are the people you know will get on board, by your side, once your new train pulls into the station.

(Change of scene: Telephone call between California and Germany. Cast: Steve, Paula, Annette, and a telephone operator/translator. Split-screen close-ups on Annette and Steve as Steve narrates.)

My Donor Now and Always

It had been just two and a half years, yet it seemed like a lifetime. In effect, it was. In the early hours of May 4, 2002, I received a bone marrow transplant at City of Hope, the aim to rid me of acute leukemia. Now healthy and back to work as a sports writer, I recently picked up the photo of me holding the "4" from the tear-off calendar as my donor's blood was fed into my body at around 3 a.m. In the photo with me was my nurse. Behind the camera at that special moment was my mom, and next to her was my grandmother. Some thousands and thousands of miles away, halfway around the world in fact, an angel stood by.

We didn't know her name, but we knew what she was all about. She was my donor, and she was there, in spirit, with us.

She had been there from the moment our doctor, David Snyder, told us she had been found.

She was close to my age, Dr. Snyder told us, around her early 30s. For legal reasons, we couldn't know anything else about her for two more years, but I didn't need to know.

I knew more about her through her incredibly unselfish deed than I had learned about others I'd known my entire life.

Yes, I saw her there with us on that early morning. Not just her blood. Her soul. It was her soul, I truly believe, that pulled me through, dragged me off the mat.

Blood is just fuel; the soul is the spirit's engine.

With my donor's "presence" and the support of those who were physically there with me, I had all the spirit I needed to rally past this supposedly devastating obstacle, this cancer.

In the days prior to the transplant, I had written my donor a letter. It was the easiest letter I'd ever written. It was from my heart. I told her that I would persevere, that her good deed would not have been done in vain. That I would, in fact, bounce back better than before.

Due to regulations that prohibit a recipient from contacting a donor, for more than two years we didn't communicate again, at least not verbally or via letter. I could not be given her address; the letter was mailed for me.

But I talked to her every day, in fact, through our souls.

The waiting period to contact a donor living outside the United States was two years from the date of the transplant.

Then came that special day. The weekend after a visit to City of Hope for a routine checkup showed I still had 100 percent healthy blood. My mom and I dialed the registry to find out my donor's whereabouts.

We told her we needed to make a call to Germany, and that we would also need a translator. (One of the early letters we received from my donor, which was screened by City of Hope, was penned in German.)

When her personal information was finally released to us, we saw that she did indeed live in Germany. We also were given more information about her than simply her first name, Annette, which we knew from her letter, just after my transplant.

We knew that she had been in the donor registry for nine years before getting word of me. Her mother had died of a brain tumor in April of 2002, she wrote in the letter (one translated for us), and she was hoping to be able to help someone else in her mother's honor.

I had been longing to thank her with my own voice.

It was 10 a.m. in Los Angeles when the call was placed. It was 7 p.m. in Germany. Annette answered the phone.

The translator was wonderful, taking an interest in our monumental conversation.

"She is on the line," the translator told me, but I knew that already because I could hear Annette's soft voice when she said hello in German. My mom listened on the phone in the other room.

The subsequent ten minutes was the easiest conversation I ever had. I spoke from the heart.

I repeated what I said in my first letter, stressing to Annette that, so far, I had held true to my promise. Then I told her how strong she was to do what she had done, donate her blood so that someone else, someone she did not know and might never meet, could live.

She replied that she only did what she had to do. My mom then thanked her as well.

As the operator translated and Annette responded in her native language, I had time to digest the magnitude of the conversation.

As wonderful as that conversation was, it was of the same magnitude as the first moment I heard she had been found.

When someone special is in your life, you know it, whether they're standing next to you or halfway across the world.

Annette will always be with me, as will Dr. Snyder, as will my mom and my grandmother, and that nurse in the photo.

All that time has passed and, thanks to Annette's coming forward to "do what she had to do," it seems like a lifetime ago.

It was because that was the day I began to live.

Thank you, Annette, now and always. I won't let you down.

(Scene change: Annette sits at a table at her home in Germany composing a note in German to Steve.)

Giving Life and Receiving Thanks

Dear Steve:

It pleases me that you are continuing to get better and can enjoy life to its fullest. It always gives me a good feeling that I was able to help you and that your transplant went so well. Thank you for the red heart you sent me. I think of you often and wish you the best.

Best wishes,

Annette

(Scene change: Paula's Los Angeles home. Close-up on Paula and she narrates. She holds a photo of a huge professional football player.)

Mom's Final Thoughts

After Steve returned to his job as a sportswriter five months after his successful transplant, he wrote a number of stories about the surprising benefits of having cancer. One was being forced to take the time to figure out what really matters in life. Relationships, he wrote, are the most important, in addition to all of his family.

Steve was lucky enough to have a terrific relationship with a fellow graduate of the University of Michigan.

Rod Payne, who played football at Michigan and went on to play four years in the NFL, winning the Super Bowl as a backup center with the 2000 Baltimore Ravens, was an unwavering source of support for Steve during his illness, not only support, but also strength and motivation to survive, as well.

They had big plans, these two, both personally and professionally. Though an unlikely team, as sportswriters and athletes usually are in today's anti-media world, they nonetheless teamed up to fight Steve's cancer together.

Steve and Rod have a book, *Centering on a Miracle*, which was published in 2006 and is available in bookstores and online. It shows what friendship, faith, family, and medical science can do when combined to save a life.

Every cancer patient, Steve told me, should be fortunate enough to have a Super Bowl champion by his or her bedside to rally him or her through the dark days.

We, Steve's family members, were always there for him, but sometimes one needs a peer, someone on an equal level emotionally.

That's what he had in Rod, a giant of a man both literally and figuratively, who picked my son up off the mat and then raised his arm in victory.

God bless you, Rod.

Epilogue

Annette traveled from Germany to meet Steve at City of Hope's Bone Marrow Transplant Survivor's Day. Steve and Rod both live in Florida and travel around the country promoting their book, *Centered by a Miracle: A True Story of Friendship, Football & Life*, and speaking about the "Healing Power of Teamwork!" Pearl passed away at age 84.

Paula continues her nursing job. Dr. Snyder keeps saving lives at City of Hope. Julie continues teaching Writing for Wellness classes at the Hope Village Comedy Theatre.

About the Author

Julie Davey has loved the written word and classrooms since she was four years old. Her late mother told about Julie slipping into the adjoining elementary school's kindergarten class for story time. To avoid detection, she hid behind the "big kids" circled around the teacher.

Julie wrote for her junior-high and high school newspapers and became editor-in-chief of the Colorado Woman's College newspaper. She received her associate's degree from CWC, her bachelor's degree in Journalism and a master's degree in American Studies from California State University, Los Angeles.

She worked as a newspaper reporter (*Laredo Times*) and television writer (*KGNS-TV*) in Laredo, Texas. She was a political reporter (*San Antonio Light)* and an associate magazine editor (*Engineering and Science)* at the California Institute of Technology.

She taught journalism and English at Glendale (CA) High School. When she became a full-time college professor at Fullerton College, she was the adviser for the campus newspaper (*The Hornet*), which won Columbia University's Gold Crown award. Julie received Fullerton College's highest award for excellence in teaching.

She is the author of a political novel, *La Caridad*, (Ashley Books 1991) and scores of newspaper and magazine articles.

In 2001, she created Writing for Wellness classes for her fellow cancer patients at City of Hope and continues to teach bi-weekly classes. In 2006 she was named "Woman of the Week" by *CBS News* in Los Angeles. City of Hope designated her as a Survivor of the Year and gave her the Heart of Hope award for her volunteer work.

She and her husband, Bob, live in Duarte, California.

She still loves the written word and her favorite classroom activity is still story time.